Goal

Getter

ISBN 978-0-6457450-0-9

Your Goal Getter Journal

This journal is designed to help you set and make the changes you want to your life.

It is designed for you to be able to start at any time so there are no specific dates and you can work to your own timetable.

The 12 Month Planner allows you to enter your main events and goals. While the Monthly Focus gives you space to break down the one or two things you really want to focus on for that month.

The Weekly Snapshot is where you plan out the week ahead and review it at the end.

I have prefilled some Quotes for the Week and others are blank for you to write your own inspirational quote.

And lastly, your Daily Plan is where you to enter the things you want to get done each day. There is a space for you to write your Biggest Learning for the day and your Magic Moment for each day. It is these small things that can really help show you how you are changing and to appreciate each day.

Use some, or all of it to help you achieve your goals.

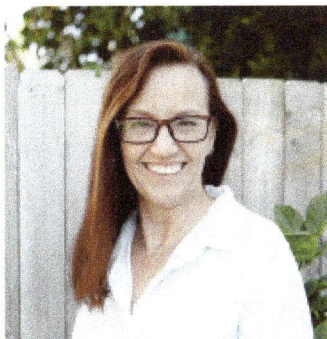

My wish for you is that using this journal helps you fulfil the goals and plans you set for yourself.

Remember all journeys start with a single step, but you need to keep putting one foot in front of the other to get to your destination.

Libby Salmon

The Big Picture

12 Month Planner

January	February	March

April	May	June

July	August	September

October	November	December

Monthly
Focus

Goals	Due By

Tasks

- [ ]
- [ ]
- [ ]
- [ ]
- [ ]
- [ ]

Results

Weekly
Snapshot

New Habit

Name It.

Must Do This Week!

Track It.

- ☐ Mon
- ☐ Tues
- ☐ Wed
- ☐ Thurs
- ☐ Fri
- ☐ Sat
- ☐ Sun

Quote For The Week:

While we are postponing,
life speeds by.
SENECA

Review It.
How did it go?
What worked?
What didn't?

Daily Plan

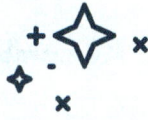

Day at a glance

6 am	
7 am	
8 am	
9 am	
10 am	
11 am	
12 pm	
1 pm	
2 pm	
3 pm	
4 pm	
5 pm	
6 pm	
7 pm	

Remember This!

Top Priorities!

Glass of Water Score

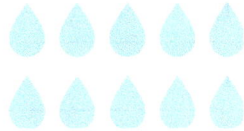

Biggest Learning:

Today's Magic Moment:

Daily
Plan

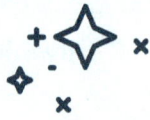

Day at a glance

6 am	
7 am	
8 am	
9 am	
10 am	
11 am	
12 pm	
1 pm	
2 pm	
3 pm	
4 pm	
5 pm	
6 pm	
7 pm	

Remember This!

Top Priorities!

Glass of Water Score

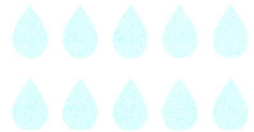

Biggest Learning:

Today's Magic Moment:

Daily

Plan

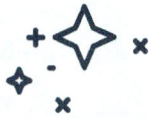

Day at a glance

6 am	
7 am	
8 am	
9 am	
10 am	
11 am	
12 pm	
1 pm	
2 pm	
3 pm	
4 pm	
5 pm	
6 pm	
7 pm	

Top Priorities!

Glass of Water Score

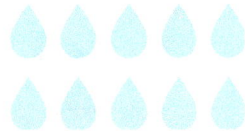

Biggest Learning:

Today's Magic Moment:

Daily
Plan

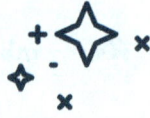

Day at a glance

6 am	
7 am	
8 am	
9 am	
10 am	
11 am	
12 pm	
1 pm	
2 pm	
3 pm	
4 pm	
5 pm	
6 pm	
7 pm	

Remember This!

Top Priorities!

Glass of Water Score

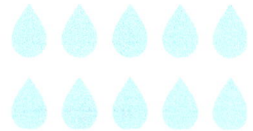

Biggest Learning:

Today's Magic Moment:

Daily Plan

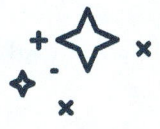

Day at a glance

Time	
6 am	
7 am	
8 am	
9 am	
10 am	
11 am	
12 pm	
1 pm	
2 pm	
3 pm	
4 pm	
5 pm	
6 pm	
7 pm	

Remember This!

Top Priorities!

Glass of Water Score

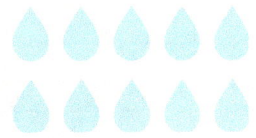

Biggest Learning:

Today's Magic Moment:

Daily Plan

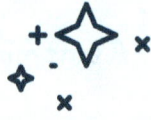

Day at a glance

Time	
6 am	
7 am	
8 am	
9 am	
10 am	
11 am	
12 pm	
1 pm	
2 pm	
3 pm	
4 pm	
5 pm	
6 pm	
7 pm	

Remember This!

Top Priorities!

Glass of Water Score

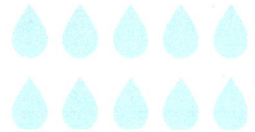

Biggest Learning:

Today's Magic Moment:

Daily Plan

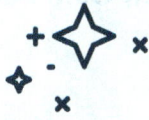

Day at a glance

6 am	
7 am	
8 am	
9 am	
10 am	
11 am	
12 pm	
1 pm	
2 pm	
3 pm	
4 pm	
5 pm	
6 pm	
7 pm	

Remember This!

Top Priorities!

Glass of Water Score

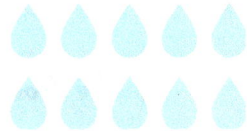

Biggest Learning:

Today's Magic Moment:

Weekly Snapshot

New Habit

Name It.

Must Do This Week!

Track It.

☐ Mon

☐ Tues

☐ Wed

☐ Thurs

☐ Fri

☐ Sat

☐ Sun

Quote For The Week:

Not all of us can do great things.

But we can do small things with great love.

MOTHER TERESA

Review It.
How did it go?
What worked?
What didn't?

Daily Plan

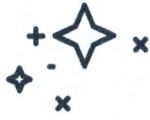

Day at a glance

6 am	
7 am	
8 am	
9 am	
10 am	
11 am	
12 pm	
1 pm	
2 pm	
3 pm	
4 pm	
5 pm	
6 pm	
7 pm	

Remember This!

Top Priorities!

Glass of Water Score

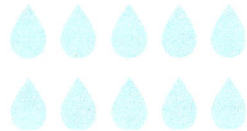

Biggest Learning:

Today's Magic Moment:

Daily
Plan

Day at a glance

6 am	
7 am	
8 am	
9 am	
10 am	
11 am	
12 pm	
1 pm	
2 pm	
3 pm	
4 pm	
5 pm	
6 pm	
7 pm	

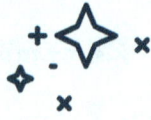

Remember This!

Top Priorities!

Glass of Water Score

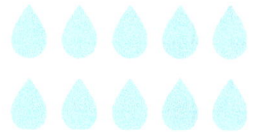

Biggest Learning:

Today's Magic Moment:

Daily Plan

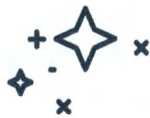

Day at a glance

6 am	
7 am	
8 am	
9 am	
10 am	
11 am	
12 pm	
1 pm	
2 pm	
3 pm	
4 pm	
5 pm	
6 pm	
7 pm	

Remember This!

Top Priorities!

Glass of Water Score

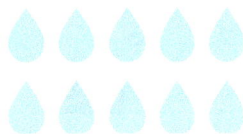

Biggest Learning:

Today's Magic Moment:

Daily
Plan

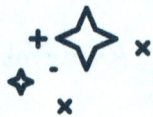

Day at a glance

6 am	
7 am	
8 am	
9 am	
10 am	
11 am	
12 pm	
1 pm	
2 pm	
3 pm	
4 pm	
5 pm	
6 pm	
7 pm	

Top Priorities!

Glass of Water Score

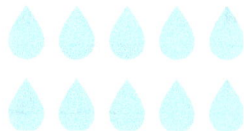

Biggest Learning:

Today's Magic Moment:

Daily Plan

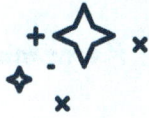

Day at a glance

Time	
6 am	
7 am	
8 am	
9 am	
10 am	
11 am	
12 pm	
1 pm	
2 pm	
3 pm	
4 pm	
5 pm	
6 pm	
7 pm	

Remember This!

Top Priorities!

Glass of Water Score

Biggest Learning:

Today's Magic Moment:

Daily Plan

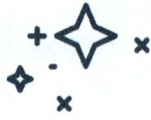

Day at a glance

Remember This!

6 am	
7 am	
8 am	
9 am	
10 am	
11 am	
12 pm	
1 pm	
2 pm	
3 pm	
4 pm	
5 pm	
6 pm	
7 pm	

Top Priorities!

Glass of Water Score

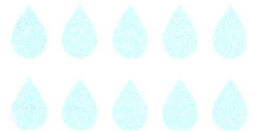

Biggest Learning:

Today's Magic Moment:

Daily Plan

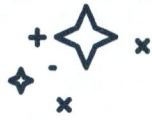

Day at a glance

6 am	
7 am	
8 am	
9 am	
10 am	
11 am	
12 pm	
1 pm	
2 pm	
3 pm	
4 pm	
5 pm	
6 pm	
7 pm	

Remember This!

Top Priorities!

Glass of Water Score

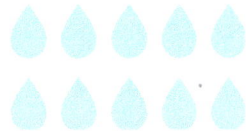

Biggest Learning:

Today's Magic Moment:

Weekly Snapshot

Week Commencing:

New Habit

Name It.

Must Do This Week!

Track It.

☐ Mon

☐ Tues

☐ Wed

☐ Thurs

☐ Fri

☐ Sat

☐ Sun

Quote For The Week:

Review It.
How did it go?
What worked?
What didn't?

Daily Plan

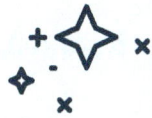

Day at a glance

6 am	
7 am	
8 am	
9 am	
10 am	
11 am	
12 pm	
1 pm	
2 pm	
3 pm	
4 pm	
5 pm	
6 pm	
7 pm	

Remember This!

Top Priorities!

Glass of Water Score

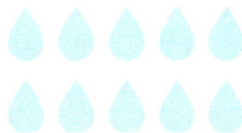

Biggest Learning:

Today's Magic Moment:

Daily
Plan
Day at a glance

6 am	
7 am	
8 am	
9 am	
10 am	
11 am	
12 pm	
1 pm	
2 pm	
3 pm	
4 pm	
5 pm	
6 pm	
7 pm	

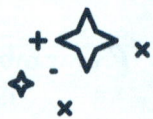

Remember This!

Top Priorities!

Glass of Water Score

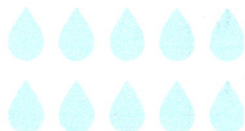

Biggest Learning:

Today's Magic Moment:

Daily
Plan

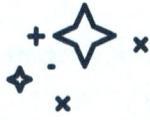

Day at a glance

6 am	
7 am	
8 am	
9 am	
10 am	
11 am	
12 pm	
1 pm	
2 pm	
3 pm	
4 pm	
5 pm	
6 pm	
7 pm	

Top Priorities!

Glass of Water Score

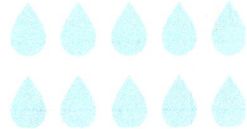

Biggest Learning:

Today's Magic Moment:

Daily Plan

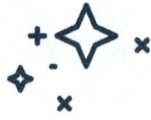

Day at a glance

6 am	
7 am	
8 am	
9 am	
10 am	
11 am	
12 pm	
1 pm	
2 pm	
3 pm	
4 pm	
5 pm	
6 pm	
7 pm	

Remember This!

Top Priorities!

Glass of Water Score

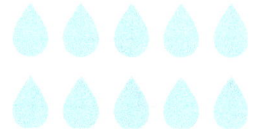

💧💧💧💧💧
💧💧💧💧💧

Biggest Learning:

Today's Magic Moment:

Daily
Plan

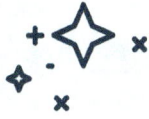

Day at a glance

6 am	
7 am	
8 am	
9 am	
10 am	
11 am	
12 pm	
1 pm	
2 pm	
3 pm	
4 pm	
5 pm	
6 pm	
7 pm	

Top Priorities!

Glass of Water Score

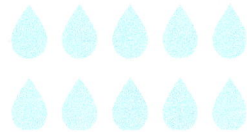

Biggest Learning:

Today's Magic Moment:

Daily Plan

Day at a glance

6 am	
7 am	
8 am	
9 am	
10 am	
11 am	
12 pm	
1 pm	
2 pm	
3 pm	
4 pm	
5 pm	
6 pm	
7 pm	

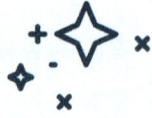

Remember This!

Top Priorities!

Glass of Water Score

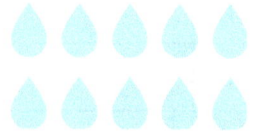

Biggest Learning:

Today's Magic Moment:

Daily Plan

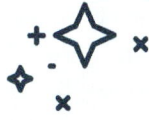

Day at a glance

6 am	
7 am	
8 am	
9 am	
10 am	
11 am	
12 pm	
1 pm	
2 pm	
3 pm	
4 pm	
5 pm	
6 pm	
7 pm	

Remember This!

Top Priorities!

Glass of Water Score

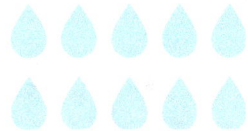

Biggest Learning:

Today's Magic Moment:

Weekly Snapshot

New Habit

Name It.

Must Do This Week!

Track It.

- ☐ Mon
- ☐ Tues
- ☐ Wed
- ☐ Thurs
- ☐ Fri
- ☐ Sat
- ☐ Sun

Quote For The Week:

Do the best you can until you know better.

Then when you know better, do better.

MAYA ANGELOU

Review It.
How did it go?
What worked?
What didn't?

Daily Plan

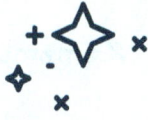

Day at a glance

6 am	
7 am	
8 am	
9 am	
10 am	
11 am	
12 pm	
1 pm	
2 pm	
3 pm	
4 pm	
5 pm	
6 pm	
7 pm	

Remember This!

Top Priorities!

Glass of Water Score

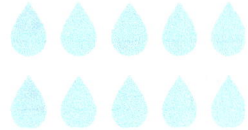

Biggest Learning:

Today's Magic Moment:

Daily
Plan

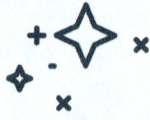

Day at a glance

Remember This!

6 am	
7 am	
8 am	
9 am	
10 am	
11 am	
12 pm	
1 pm	
2 pm	
3 pm	
4 pm	
5 pm	
6 pm	
7 pm	

Top Priorities!

Glass of Water Score

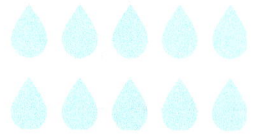

Biggest Learning:

Today's Magic Moment:

Daily Plan

Remember This! 👆

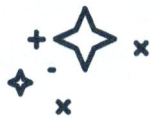

Day at a glance

6 am	
7 am	
8 am	
9 am	
10 am	
11 am	
12 pm	
1 pm	
2 pm	
3 pm	
4 pm	
5 pm	
6 pm	
7 pm	

Top Priorities!

Glass of Water Score

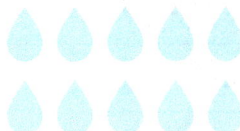

💧💧💧💧💧
💧💧💧💧💧

Biggest Learning:

Today's Magic Moment:

Daily Plan

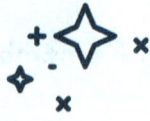

Day at a glance

6 am	
7 am	
8 am	
9 am	
10 am	
11 am	
12 pm	
1 pm	
2 pm	
3 pm	
4 pm	
5 pm	
6 pm	
7 pm	

Remember This!

Top Priorities!

Glass of Water Score

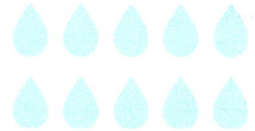

Biggest Learning:

Today's Magic Moment:

Daily

Plan

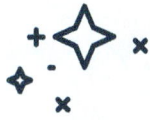

Day at a glance

6 am	
7 am	
8 am	
9 am	
10 am	
11 am	
12 pm	
1 pm	
2 pm	
3 pm	
4 pm	
5 pm	
6 pm	
7 pm	

Remember This!

Top Priorities!

Glass of Water Score

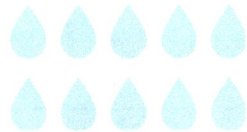

Biggest Learning:

Today's Magic Moment:

Daily Plan

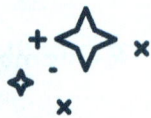

Day at a glance

Time	
6 am	
7 am	
8 am	
9 am	
10 am	
11 am	
12 pm	
1 pm	
2 pm	
3 pm	
4 pm	
5 pm	
6 pm	
7 pm	

Remember This!

Top Priorities!

Glass of Water Score

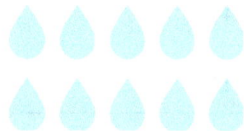

Biggest Learning:

Today's Magic Moment:

Daily
Plan

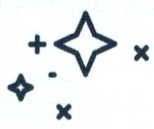

Day at a glance

6 am	
7 am	
8 am	
9 am	
10 am	
11 am	
12 pm	
1 pm	
2 pm	
3 pm	
4 pm	
5 pm	
6 pm	
7 pm	

Remember This!

Top Priorities!

Glass of Water Score

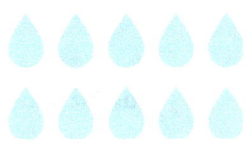

Biggest Learning:

Today's Magic Moment:

Weekly
Snapshot

Week Commencing:

Must Do This Week!

New Habit
Name It.

Track It.

☐ Mon

☐ Tues

☐ Wed

☐ Thurs

☐ Fri

☐ Sat

☐ Sun

Quote For The Week:

Review It.
How did it go?
What worked?
What didn't?

Daily Plan

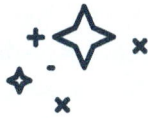

Day at a glance

6 am	
7 am	
8 am	
9 am	
10 am	
11 am	
12 pm	
1 pm	
2 pm	
3 pm	
4 pm	
5 pm	
6 pm	
7 pm	

Remember This!

Top Priorities!

Glass of Water Score

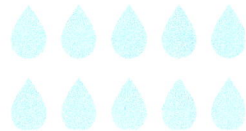

Biggest Learning:

Today's Magic Moment:

Daily
Plan
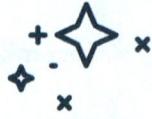

Day at a glance

Remember This!

6 am	
7 am	
8 am	
9 am	
10 am	
11 am	
12 pm	
1 pm	
2 pm	
3 pm	
4 pm	
5 pm	
6 pm	
7 pm	

Top Priorities!

Glass of Water Score

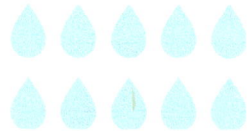

Biggest Learning:

Today's Magic Moment:

Daily Plan

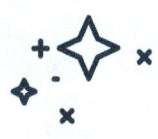

Day at a glance

6 am	
7 am	
8 am	
9 am	
10 am	
11 am	
12 pm	
1 pm	
2 pm	
3 pm	
4 pm	
5 pm	
6 pm	
7 pm	

Remember This!

Top Priorities!

Glass of Water Score

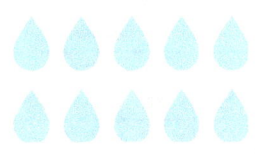

Biggest Learning:

Today's Magic Moment:

Daily
Plan

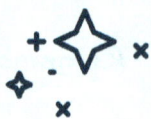

Day at a glance

6 am	
7 am	
8 am	
9 am	
10 am	
11 am	
12 pm	
1 pm	
2 pm	
3 pm	
4 pm	
5 pm	
6 pm	
7 pm	

Top Priorities!

Glass of Water Score

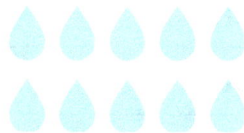

💧💧💧💧💧
💧💧💧💧💧

Biggest Learning:

Today's Magic Moment:

Daily Plan

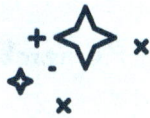

Day at a glance

6 am	
7 am	
8 am	
9 am	
10 am	
11 am	
12 pm	
1 pm	
2 pm	
3 pm	
4 pm	
5 pm	
6 pm	
7 pm	

Remember This!

Top Priorities!

Glass of Water Score

Biggest Learning:

Today's Magic Moment:

Daily Plan

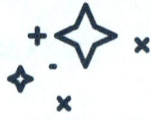

Day at a glance

6 am	
7 am	
8 am	
9 am	
10 am	
11 am	
12 pm	
1 pm	
2 pm	
3 pm	
4 pm	
5 pm	
6 pm	
7 pm	

Remember This!

Top Priorities!

Glass of Water Score

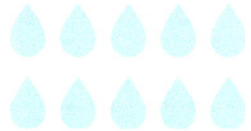

Biggest Learning:

Today's Magic Moment:

Daily Plan

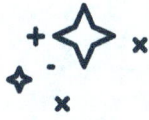

Day at a glance

6 am	
7 am	
8 am	
9 am	
10 am	
11 am	
12 pm	
1 pm	
2 pm	
3 pm	
4 pm	
5 pm	
6 pm	
7 pm	

Remember This!

Top Priorities!

Glass of Water Score

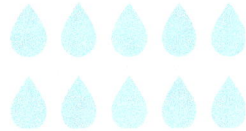

Biggest Learning:

Today's Magic Moment:

Monthly
Focus

Goals	Due By

Results

Tasks

- [ ]
- [ ]
- [ ]
- [ ]
- [ ]
- [ ]

Weekly Snapshot

Week Commencing:

New Habit

Name It.

Must Do This Week!

Track It.

- [ ] Mon
- [ ] Tues
- [ ] Wed
- [ ] Thurs
- [ ] Fri
- [ ] Sat
- [ ] Sun

Quote For The Week:

Watch your thoughts;
they become words.
Watch your words;
they become actions.
Watch your actions;
they become habits.
Watch your habits;
they become character.
Watch your character;
it becomes your destiny.
LAO TZU

Review It.

How did it go?
What worked?
What didn't?

Daily
Plan

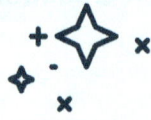

Day at a glance

Remember This!

6 am	
7 am	
8 am	
9 am	
10 am	
11 am	
12 pm	
1 pm	
2 pm	
3 pm	
4 pm	
5 pm	
6 pm	
7 pm	

Top Priorities!

Glass of Water Score

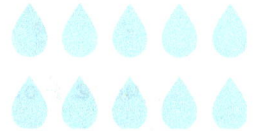

Biggest Learning:

Today's Magic Moment:

Daily Plan

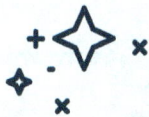

Day at a glance

6 am	
7 am	
8 am	
9 am	
10 am	
11 am	
12 pm	
1 pm	
2 pm	
3 pm	
4 pm	
5 pm	
6 pm	
7 pm	

Remember This!

Top Priorities!

Glass of Water Score

Biggest Learning:

Today's Magic Moment:

Daily Plan

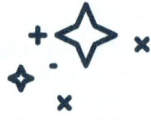

Day at a glance

6 am	
7 am	
8 am	
9 am	
10 am	
11 am	
12 pm	
1 pm	
2 pm	
3 pm	
4 pm	
5 pm	
6 pm	
7 pm	

Remember This!

Top Priorities!

Glass of Water Score

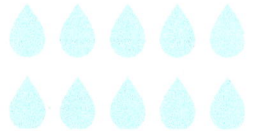

Biggest Learning:

Today's Magic Moment:

Daily Plan

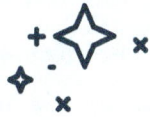

Day at a glance

Remember This!

6 am	
7 am	
8 am	
9 am	
10 am	
11 am	
12 pm	
1 pm	
2 pm	
3 pm	
4 pm	
5 pm	
6 pm	
7 pm	

Top Priorities!

Glass of Water Score

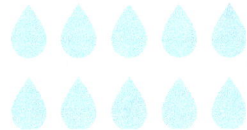

Biggest Learning:

Today's Magic Moment:

Daily Plan

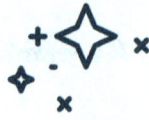

Day at a glance

6 am	
7 am	
8 am	
9 am	
10 am	
11 am	
12 pm	
1 pm	
2 pm	
3 pm	
4 pm	
5 pm	
6 pm	
7 pm	

Top Priorities!

Glass of Water Score

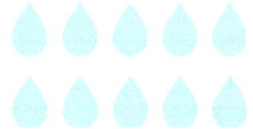

Biggest Learning:

Today's Magic Moment:

Daily Plan

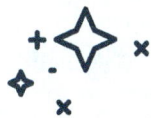

Day at a glance

6 am	
7 am	
8 am	
9 am	
10 am	
11 am	
12 pm	
1 pm	
2 pm	
3 pm	
4 pm	
5 pm	
6 pm	
7 pm	

Remember This!

Top Priorities!

Glass of Water Score

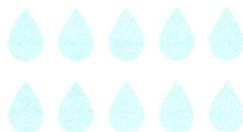

Biggest Learning:

Today's Magic Moment:

Daily Plan

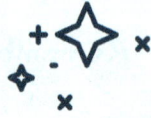

Day at a glance

6 am	
7 am	
8 am	
9 am	
10 am	
11 am	
12 pm	
1 pm	
2 pm	
3 pm	
4 pm	
5 pm	
6 pm	
7 pm	

Remember This!

Top Priorities!

Glass of Water Score

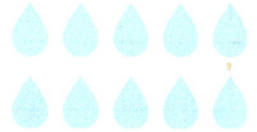

Biggest Learning:

Today's Magic Moment:

Weekly Snapshot

Week Commencing:

New Habit
Name It.

Must Do This Week!

Track It.

- ☐ Mon
- ☐ Tues
- ☐ Wed
- ☐ Thurs
- ☐ Fri
- ☐ Sat
- ☐ Sun

Quote For The Week:

Review It.
How did it go?
What worked?
What didn't?

Daily Plan

Day at a glance

6 am	
7 am	
8 am	
9 am	
10 am	
11 am	
12 pm	
1 pm	
2 pm	
3 pm	
4 pm	
5 pm	
6 pm	
7 pm	

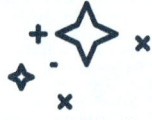

Remember This!

Top Priorities!

Glass of Water Score

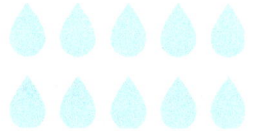

Biggest Learning:

Today's Magic Moment:

Daily
Plan

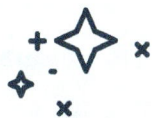

Day at a glance

6 am	
7 am	
8 am	
9 am	
10 am	
11 am	
12 pm	
1 pm	
2 pm	
3 pm	
4 pm	
5 pm	
6 pm	
7 pm	

Remember This!

Top Priorities!

Glass of Water Score

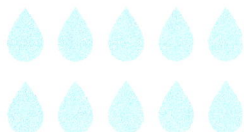

Biggest Learning:

Today's Magic Moment:

Daily Plan

Day at a glance

Time	
6 am	
7 am	
8 am	
9 am	
10 am	
11 am	
12 pm	
1 pm	
2 pm	
3 pm	
4 pm	
5 pm	
6 pm	
7 pm	

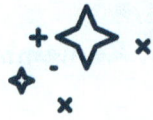

Remember This!

Top Priorities!

Glass of Water Score

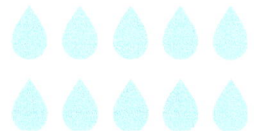

Biggest Learning:

Today's Magic Moment:

Daily

Plan

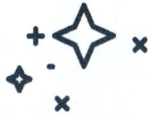

Day at a glance

6 am	
7 am	
8 am	
9 am	
10 am	
11 am	
12 pm	
1 pm	
2 pm	
3 pm	
4 pm	
5 pm	
6 pm	
7 pm	

Remember This!

Top Priorities!

Glass of Water Score

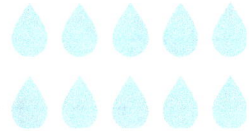

Biggest Learning:

Today's Magic Moment:

Daily Plan

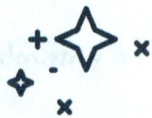

Day at a glance

6 am	
7 am	
8 am	
9 am	
10 am	
11 am	
12 pm	
1 pm	
2 pm	
3 pm	
4 pm	
5 pm	
6 pm	
7 pm	

Remember This!

Top Priorities!

Glass of Water Score

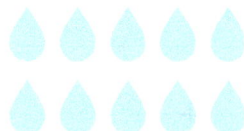

Biggest Learning:

Today's Magic Moment:

Daily
Plan

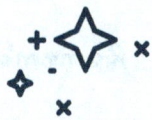

Day at a glance

Time	
6 am	
7 am	
8 am	
9 am	
10 am	
11 am	
12 pm	
1 pm	
2 pm	
3 pm	
4 pm	
5 pm	
6 pm	
7 pm	

Remember This!

Top Priorities!

Glass of Water Score

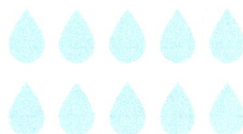

Biggest Learning:

Today's Magic Moment:

Daily Plan

Day at a glance

6 am	
7 am	
8 am	
9 am	
10 am	
11 am	
12 pm	
1 pm	
2 pm	
3 pm	
4 pm	
5 pm	
6 pm	
7 pm	

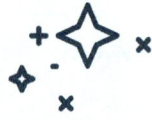

Remember This!

Top Priorities!

Glass of Water Score

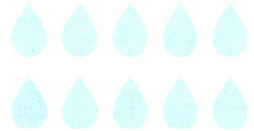

Biggest Learning:

Today's Magic Moment:

Weekly Snapshot

Week Commencing:

Must Do This Week!

New Habit

Name It.

Track It.

- ☐ Mon
- ☐ Tues
- ☐ Wed
- ☐ Thurs
- ☐ Fri
- ☐ Sat
- ☐ Sun

Quote For The Week:

Do the thing you think you cannot do.

ELEANOR ROOSEVELT

Review It.
How did it go?
What worked?
What didn't?

Daily Plan

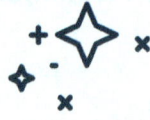

Day at a glance

Time	
6 am	
7 am	
8 am	
9 am	
10 am	
11 am	
12 pm	
1 pm	
2 pm	
3 pm	
4 pm	
5 pm	
6 pm	
7 pm	

Remember This!

Top Priorities!

Glass of Water Score

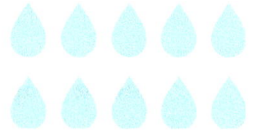

Biggest Learning:

Today's Magic Moment:

Daily
Plan

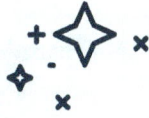

Day at a glance

6 am	
7 am	
8 am	
9 am	
10 am	
11 am	
12 pm	
1 pm	
2 pm	
3 pm	
4 pm	
5 pm	
6 pm	
7 pm	

Top Priorities!

Glass of Water Score

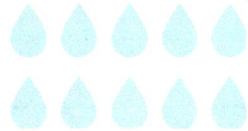

Biggest Learning:

Today's Magic Moment:

Daily Plan

Day at a glance

6 am	
7 am	
8 am	
9 am	
10 am	
11 am	
12 pm	
1 pm	
2 pm	
3 pm	
4 pm	
5 pm	
6 pm	
7 pm	

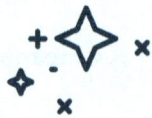

Remember This!

Top Priorities!

Glass of Water Score

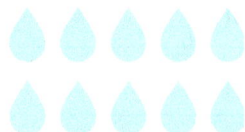

Biggest Learning:

Today's Magic Moment:

Daily
Plan

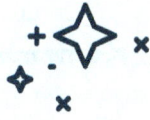

Day at a glance

Time	
6 am	
7 am	
8 am	
9 am	
10 am	
11 am	
12 pm	
1 pm	
2 pm	
3 pm	
4 pm	
5 pm	
6 pm	
7 pm	

Remember This!

Top Priorities!

Glass of Water Score

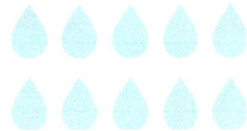

Biggest Learning:

Today's Magic Moment:

Daily Plan

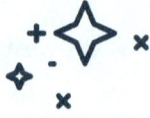

Day at a glance

6 am	
7 am	
8 am	
9 am	
10 am	
11 am	
12 pm	
1 pm	
2 pm	
3 pm	
4 pm	
5 pm	
6 pm	
7 pm	

Remember This!

Top Priorities!

Glass of Water Score

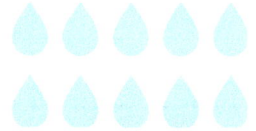

Biggest Learning:

Today's Magic Moment:

Daily
Plan

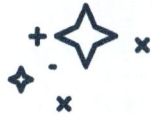

Day at a glance

6 am	
7 am	
8 am	
9 am	
10 am	
11 am	
12 pm	
1 pm	
2 pm	
3 pm	
4 pm	
5 pm	
6 pm	
7 pm	

Remember This!

Top Priorities!

Glass of Water Score

Biggest Learning:

Today's Magic Moment:

Daily
Plan

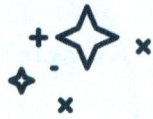

Day at a glance

6 am	
7 am	
8 am	
9 am	
10 am	
11 am	
12 pm	
1 pm	
2 pm	
3 pm	
4 pm	
5 pm	
6 pm	
7 pm	

Top Priorities!

Glass of Water Score

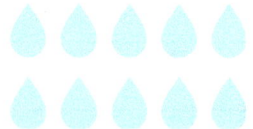

💧💧💧💧💧
💧💧💧💧💧

Biggest Learning:

Today's Magic Moment:

Weekly Snapshot

Week Commencing:

New Habit

Name It.

Must Do This Week!

Track It.

- ☐ Mon
- ☐ Tues
- ☐ Wed
- ☐ Thurs
- ☐ Fri
- ☐ Sat
- ☐ Sun

Quote For The Week:

Review It.
How did it go?
What worked?
What didn't?

Daily Plan

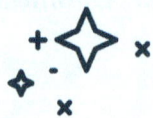

Day at a glance

6 am	
7 am	
8 am	
9 am	
10 am	
11 am	
12 pm	
1 pm	
2 pm	
3 pm	
4 pm	
5 pm	
6 pm	
7 pm	

Top Priorities!

Glass of Water Score

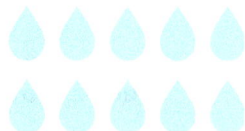

Biggest Learning:

Today's Magic Moment:

Daily Plan

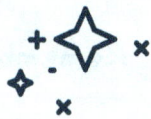

Day at a glance

6 am	
7 am	
8 am	
9 am	
10 am	
11 am	
12 pm	
1 pm	
2 pm	
3 pm	
4 pm	
5 pm	
6 pm	
7 pm	

Top Priorities!

Glass of Water Score

Biggest Learning:

Today's Magic Moment:

Daily Plan

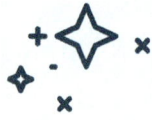

Day at a glance

Time	
6 am	
7 am	
8 am	
9 am	
10 am	
11 am	
12 pm	
1 pm	
2 pm	
3 pm	
4 pm	
5 pm	
6 pm	
7 pm	

Remember This!

Top Priorities!

Glass of Water Score

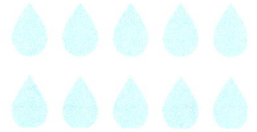

Biggest Learning:

Today's Magic Moment:

Daily Plan

Day at a glance

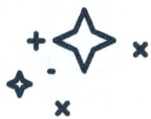

Remember This!

Time	
6 am	
7 am	
8 am	
9 am	
10 am	
11 am	
12 pm	
1 pm	
2 pm	
3 pm	
4 pm	
5 pm	
6 pm	
7 pm	

Top Priorities!

Glass of Water Score

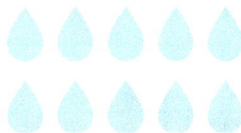

Biggest Learning:

Today's Magic Moment:

Daily Plan

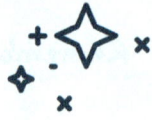

Day at a glance

6 am	
7 am	
8 am	
9 am	
10 am	
11 am	
12 pm	
1 pm	
2 pm	
3 pm	
4 pm	
5 pm	
6 pm	
7 pm	

Remember This!

Top Priorities!

Glass of Water Score

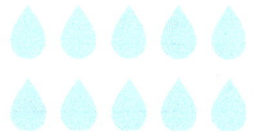

Biggest Learning:

Today's Magic Moment:

Daily
Plan

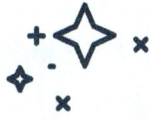

Day at a glance

6 am	
7 am	
8 am	
9 am	
10 am	
11 am	
12 pm	
1 pm	
2 pm	
3 pm	
4 pm	
5 pm	
6 pm	
7 pm	

Top Priorities!

Glass of Water Score

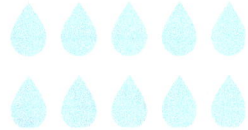

Biggest Learning:

Today's Magic Moment:

Daily Plan

Day at a glance

6 am	
7 am	
8 am	
9 am	
10 am	
11 am	
12 pm	
1 pm	
2 pm	
3 pm	
4 pm	
5 pm	
6 pm	
7 pm	

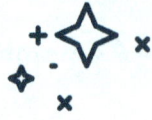

Remember This!

Top Priorities!

Glass of Water Score

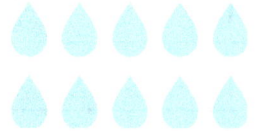

Biggest Learning:

Today's Magic Moment:

Weekly Snapshot

Week Commencing:

New Habit

Name It.

Must Do This Week!

Track It.

- ☐ Mon
- ☐ Tues
- ☐ Wed
- ☐ Thurs
- ☐ Fri
- ☐ Sat
- ☐ Sun

Quote For The Week:

Today's accomplishments
were yesterday's
impossibilities.

ROBERT SCHULLER

Review It.
How did it go?
What worked?
What didn't?

Daily Plan

Day at a glance

6 am	
7 am	
8 am	
9 am	
10 am	
11 am	
12 pm	
1 pm	
2 pm	
3 pm	
4 pm	
5 pm	
6 pm	
7 pm	

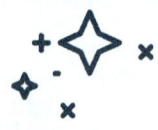

Remember This!

Top Priorities!

Glass of Water Score

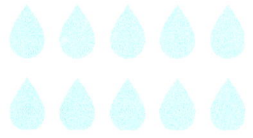

Biggest Learning:

Today's Magic Moment:

Daily Plan

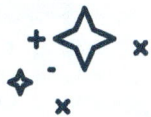

Day at a glance

6 am	
7 am	
8 am	
9 am	
10 am	
11 am	
12 pm	
1 pm	
2 pm	
3 pm	
4 pm	
5 pm	
6 pm	
7 pm	

Remember This!

Top Priorities!

Glass of Water Score

Biggest Learning:

Today's Magic Moment:

Daily Plan

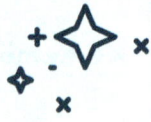

Day at a glance

Remember This!

6 am	
7 am	
8 am	
9 am	
10 am	
11 am	
12 pm	
1 pm	
2 pm	
3 pm	
4 pm	
5 pm	
6 pm	
7 pm	

Top Priorities!

Glass of Water Score

Biggest Learning:

Today's Magic Moment:

Daily Plan

Day at a glance

6 am	
7 am	
8 am	
9 am	
10 am	
11 am	
12 pm	
1 pm	
2 pm	
3 pm	
4 pm	
5 pm	
6 pm	
7 pm	

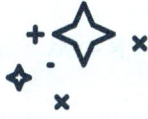

Remember This!

Top Priorities!

Glass of Water Score

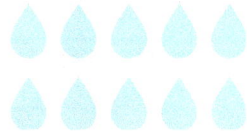

Biggest Learning:

Today's Magic Moment:

Daily Plan

Day at a glance

6 am	
7 am	
8 am	
9 am	
10 am	
11 am	
12 pm	
1 pm	
2 pm	
3 pm	
4 pm	
5 pm	
6 pm	
7 pm	

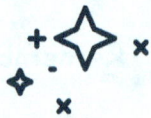

Remember This!

Top Priorities!

Glass of Water Score

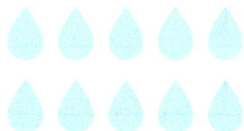

Biggest Learning:

Today's Magic Moment:

Daily

Plan

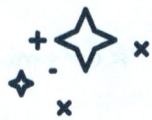

Day at a glance

6 am	
7 am	
8 am	
9 am	
10 am	
11 am	
12 pm	
1 pm	
2 pm	
3 pm	
4 pm	
5 pm	
6 pm	
7 pm	

Remember This!

Top Priorities!

Glass of Water Score

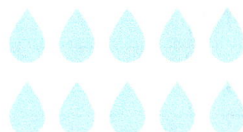

Biggest Learning:

Today's Magic Moment:

Daily
Plan
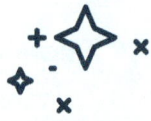

Day at a glance

Remember This!

6 am	
7 am	
8 am	
9 am	
10 am	
11 am	
12 pm	
1 pm	
2 pm	
3 pm	
4 pm	
5 pm	
6 pm	
7 pm	

Top Priorities!

Glass of Water Score

Biggest Learning:

Today's Magic Moment:

Monthly

Focus

Goals	Due By

Results

Tasks

- [ ]
- [ ]
- [ ]
- [ ]
- [ ]
- [ ]

Weekly Snapshot

Week Commencing:

Must Do This Week!

New Habit

Name It.

Track It.

- ☐ Mon
- ☐ Tues
- ☐ Wed
- ☐ Thurs
- ☐ Fri
- ☐ Sat
- ☐ Sun

Quote For The Week:

Review It.

How did it go?
What worked?
What didn't?

Daily
Plan

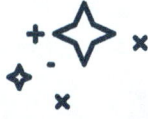

Day at a glance

6 am	
7 am	
8 am	
9 am	
10 am	
11 am	
12 pm	
1 pm	
2 pm	
3 pm	
4 pm	
5 pm	
6 pm	
7 pm	

Top Priorities!

Glass of Water Score

💧💧💧💧💧
💧💧💧💧💧

Biggest Learning:

Today's Magic Moment:

Daily Plan

Day at a glance

6 am	
7 am	
8 am	
9 am	
10 am	
11 am	
12 pm	
1 pm	
2 pm	
3 pm	
4 pm	
5 pm	
6 pm	
7 pm	

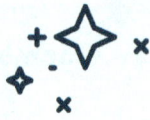

Remember This!

Top Priorities!

Glass of Water Score

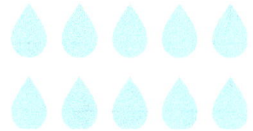

Biggest Learning:

Today's Magic Moment:

Daily Plan

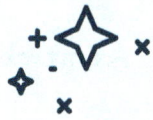

Day at a glance

Time	
6 am	
7 am	
8 am	
9 am	
10 am	
11 am	
12 pm	
1 pm	
2 pm	
3 pm	
4 pm	
5 pm	
6 pm	
7 pm	

Remember This!

Top Priorities!

Glass of Water Score

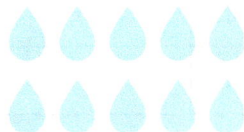

Biggest Learning:

Today's Magic Moment:

Daily Plan

Day at a glance

6 am	
7 am	
8 am	
9 am	
10 am	
11 am	
12 pm	
1 pm	
2 pm	
3 pm	
4 pm	
5 pm	
6 pm	
7 pm	

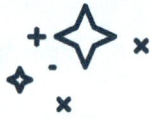

Remember This!

Top Priorities!

Glass of Water Score

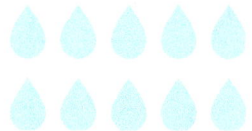

Biggest Learning:

Today's Magic Moment:

Daily Plan

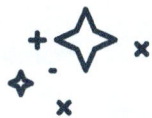

Day at a glance

6 am	
7 am	
8 am	
9 am	
10 am	
11 am	
12 pm	
1 pm	
2 pm	
3 pm	
4 pm	
5 pm	
6 pm	
7 pm	

Remember This!

Top Priorities!

Glass of Water Score

Biggest Learning:

Today's Magic Moment:

Daily Plan

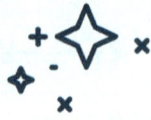

Day at a glance

6 am	
7 am	
8 am	
9 am	
10 am	
11 am	
12 pm	
1 pm	
2 pm	
3 pm	
4 pm	
5 pm	
6 pm	
7 pm	

Top Priorities!

Glass of Water Score

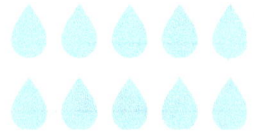

Biggest Learning:

Today's Magic Moment:

Daily

Plan

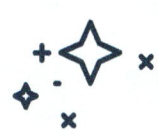

Day at a glance

6 am	
7 am	
8 am	
9 am	
10 am	
11 am	
12 pm	
1 pm	
2 pm	
3 pm	
4 pm	
5 pm	
6 pm	
7 pm	

Top Priorities!

Glass of Water Score

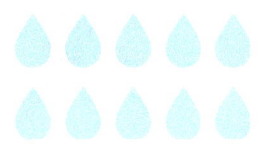

Biggest Learning:

Today's Magic Moment:

Weekly Snapshot

Week Commencing:

New Habit

Name It.

Must Do This Week!

Track It.

- ☐ Mon
- ☐ Tues
- ☐ Wed
- ☐ Thurs
- ☐ Fri
- ☐ Sat
- ☐ Sun

Quote For The Week:

Enthusiasm is the yeast that makes your hopes shine to the stars.

Enthusiasm is the sparkle in your eyes, the swing in your gait.

The grip of your hand, the irresistible surge of will and energy to execute your ideas.

HENRY FORD

Review It.

How did it go?
What worked?
What didn't?

Daily Plan

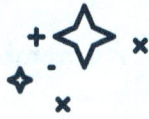

Day at a glance

6 am	
7 am	
8 am	
9 am	
10 am	
11 am	
12 pm	
1 pm	
2 pm	
3 pm	
4 pm	
5 pm	
6 pm	
7 pm	

Remember This!

Top Priorities!

Glass of Water Score

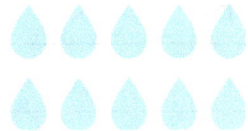

Biggest Learning:

Today's Magic Moment:

Daily Plan

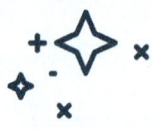

Day at a glance

6 am	
7 am	
8 am	
9 am	
10 am	
11 am	
12 pm	
1 pm	
2 pm	
3 pm	
4 pm	
5 pm	
6 pm	
7 pm	

Remember This!

Top Priorities!

Glass of Water Score

Biggest Learning:

Today's Magic Moment:

Daily
Plan

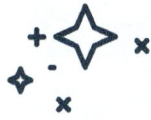

Day at a glance

6 am	
7 am	
8 am	
9 am	
10 am	
11 am	
12 pm	
1 pm	
2 pm	
3 pm	
4 pm	
5 pm	
6 pm	
7 pm	

Top Priorities!

Glass of Water Score

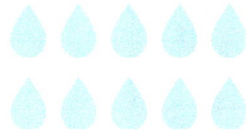

Biggest Learning:

Today's Magic Moment:

Daily Plan

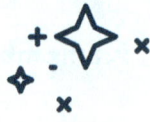

Day at a glance

Time	
6 am	
7 am	
8 am	
9 am	
10 am	
11 am	
12 pm	
1 pm	
2 pm	
3 pm	
4 pm	
5 pm	
6 pm	
7 pm	

Remember This!

Top Priorities!

Glass of Water Score

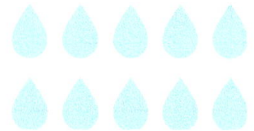

Biggest Learning:

Today's Magic Moment:

Daily Plan

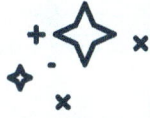

Day at a glance

6 am	
7 am	
8 am	
9 am	
10 am	
11 am	
12 pm	
1 pm	
2 pm	
3 pm	
4 pm	
5 pm	
6 pm	
7 pm	

Remember This!

Top Priorities!

Glass of Water Score

Biggest Learning:

Today's Magic Moment:

Daily Plan

Day at a glance

6 am	
7 am	
8 am	
9 am	
10 am	
11 am	
12 pm	
1 pm	
2 pm	
3 pm	
4 pm	
5 pm	
6 pm	
7 pm	

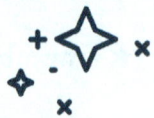

Remember This!

Top Priorities!

Glass of Water Score

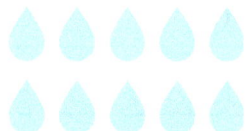

Biggest Learning:

Today's Magic Moment:

Daily Plan

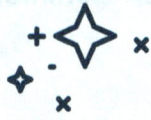

Day at a glance

6 am	
7 am	
8 am	
9 am	
10 am	
11 am	
12 pm	
1 pm	
2 pm	
3 pm	
4 pm	
5 pm	
6 pm	
7 pm	

Remember This!

Top Priorities!

Glass of Water Score

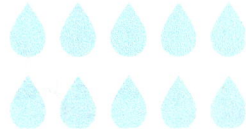

Biggest Learning:

Today's Magic Moment:

Weekly Snapshot

Week Commencing:

New Habit

Name It.

Must Do This Week!

Track It.

- ☐ Mon
- ☐ Tues
- ☐ Wed
- ☐ Thurs
- ☐ Fri
- ☐ Sat
- ☐ Sun

Quote For The Week:

Review It.
How did it go?
What worked?
What didn't?

Daily Plan

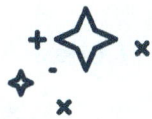

Day at a glance

6 am	
7 am	
8 am	
9 am	
10 am	
11 am	
12 pm	
1 pm	
2 pm	
3 pm	
4 pm	
5 pm	
6 pm	
7 pm	

Remember This!

Top Priorities!

Glass of Water Score

Biggest Learning:

Today's Magic Moment:

Daily
Plan
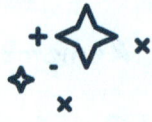

Day at a glance

Remember This!

6 am	
7 am	
8 am	
9 am	
10 am	
11 am	
12 pm	
1 pm	
2 pm	
3 pm	
4 pm	
5 pm	
6 pm	
7 pm	

Top Priorities!

Glass of Water Score

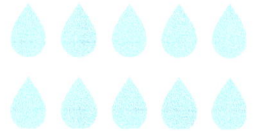

Biggest Learning:

Today's Magic Moment:

Daily Plan

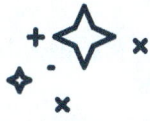

Day at a glance

6 am	
7 am	
8 am	
9 am	
10 am	
11 am	
12 pm	
1 pm	
2 pm	
3 pm	
4 pm	
5 pm	
6 pm	
7 pm	

Remember This!

Top Priorities!

Glass of Water Score

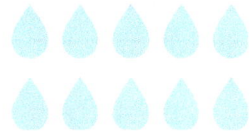

Biggest Learning:

Today's Magic Moment:

Daily Plan

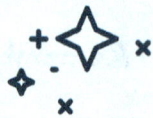

Day at a glance

6 am	
7 am	
8 am	
9 am	
10 am	
11 am	
12 pm	
1 pm	
2 pm	
3 pm	
4 pm	
5 pm	
6 pm	
7 pm	

Remember This!

Top Priorities!

Glass of Water Score

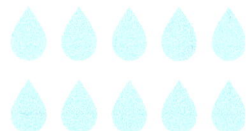

Biggest Learning:

Today's Magic Moment:

Daily Plan

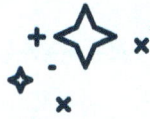

Day at a glance

Time	
6 am	
7 am	
8 am	
9 am	
10 am	
11 am	
12 pm	
1 pm	
2 pm	
3 pm	
4 pm	
5 pm	
6 pm	
7 pm	

Remember This!

Top Priorities!

Glass of Water Score

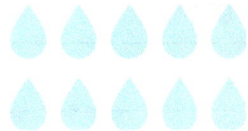

Biggest Learning:

Today's Magic Moment:

Daily Plan

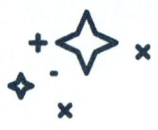

Day at a glance

6 am	
7 am	
8 am	
9 am	
10 am	
11 am	
12 pm	
1 pm	
2 pm	
3 pm	
4 pm	
5 pm	
6 pm	
7 pm	

Top Priorities!

Glass of Water Score

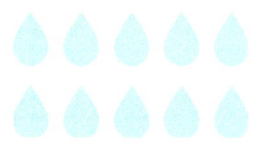

Biggest Learning:

Today's Magic Moment:

Daily Plan

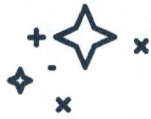

Day at a glance

6 am	
7 am	
8 am	
9 am	
10 am	
11 am	
12 pm	
1 pm	
2 pm	
3 pm	
4 pm	
5 pm	
6 pm	
7 pm	

Remember This!

Top Priorities!

Glass of Water Score

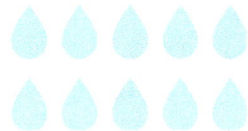

Biggest Learning:

Today's Magic Moment:

Weekly Snapshot

Week Commencing:

Must Do This Week!

New Habit

Name It.

Track It.

- ☐ Mon
- ☐ Tues
- ☐ Wed
- ☐ Thurs
- ☐ Fri
- ☐ Sat
- ☐ Sun

Quote For The Week:

We are what we repeatedly do.

Excellence, then, is not an act,
but a habit.

ARISTOTLE

Review It.
How did it go?
What worked?
What didn't?

Daily
Plan

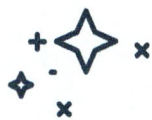

Day at a glance

Remember This!

6 am	
7 am	
8 am	
9 am	
10 am	
11 am	
12 pm	
1 pm	
2 pm	
3 pm	
4 pm	
5 pm	
6 pm	
7 pm	

Top Priorities!

Glass of Water Score

Biggest Learning:

Today's Magic Moment:

Daily Plan

Day at a glance

6 am	
7 am	
8 am	
9 am	
10 am	
11 am	
12 pm	
1 pm	
2 pm	
3 pm	
4 pm	
5 pm	
6 pm	
7 pm	

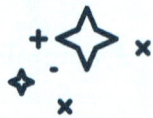

Remember This!

Top Priorities!

Glass of Water Score

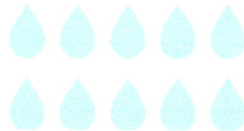

Biggest Learning:

Today's Magic Moment:

Daily Plan

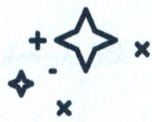

Day at a glance

6 am	
7 am	
8 am	
9 am	
10 am	
11 am	
12 pm	
1 pm	
2 pm	
3 pm	
4 pm	
5 pm	
6 pm	
7 pm	

Remember This!

Top Priorities!

Glass of Water Score

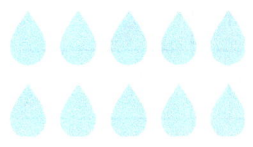

Biggest Learning:

Today's Magic Moment:

Daily
Plan
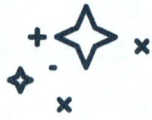

Day at a glance

Time	
6 am	
7 am	
8 am	
9 am	
10 am	
11 am	
12 pm	
1 pm	
2 pm	
3 pm	
4 pm	
5 pm	
6 pm	
7 pm	

Remember This!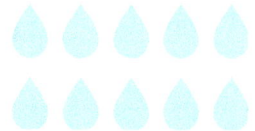

Top Priorities!

Glass of Water Score

Biggest Learning:

Today's Magic Moment:

Daily
Plan

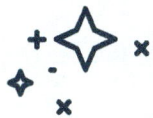

Day at a glance

6 am	
7 am	
8 am	
9 am	
10 am	
11 am	
12 pm	
1 pm	
2 pm	
3 pm	
4 pm	
5 pm	
6 pm	
7 pm	

Top Priorities!

Glass of Water Score

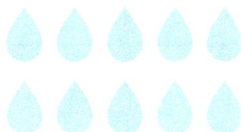

Biggest Learning:

Today's Magic Moment:

Daily Plan

Remember This!

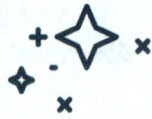

Day at a glance

6 am	
7 am	
8 am	
9 am	
10 am	
11 am	
12 pm	
1 pm	
2 pm	
3 pm	
4 pm	
5 pm	
6 pm	
7 pm	

Top Priorities!

Glass of Water Score

Biggest Learning:

Today's Magic Moment:

Daily
Plan

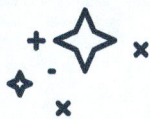

Day at a glance

6 am	
7 am	
8 am	
9 am	
10 am	
11 am	
12 pm	
1 pm	
2 pm	
3 pm	
4 pm	
5 pm	
6 pm	
7 pm	

Remember This!

Top Priorities!

Glass of Water Score

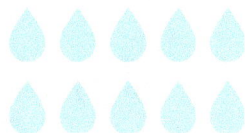

Biggest Learning:

Today's Magic Moment:

Weekly Snapshot

Week Commencing:

Must Do This Week!

New Habit

Name It.

Track It.

- ☐ Mon
- ☐ Tues
- ☐ Wed
- ☐ Thurs
- ☐ Fri
- ☐ Sat
- ☐ Sun

Quote For The Week:

Live in the present
and make it so beautiful that
it's worth remembering.

ARNOLD H. GLASOW

Review It.
How did it go?
What worked?
What didn't?

Daily Plan

Day at a glance

6 am	
7 am	
8 am	
9 am	
10 am	
11 am	
12 pm	
1 pm	
2 pm	
3 pm	
4 pm	
5 pm	
6 pm	
7 pm	

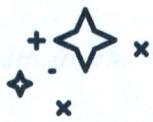

Remember This!

Top Priorities!

Glass of Water Score

Biggest Learning:

Today's Magic Moment:

Daily
Plan

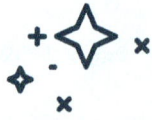

Day at a glance

6 am	
7 am	
8 am	
9 am	
10 am	
11 am	
12 pm	
1 pm	
2 pm	
3 pm	
4 pm	
5 pm	
6 pm	
7 pm	

Top Priorities!

Glass of Water Score

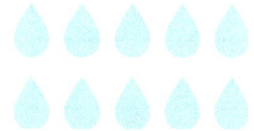

Biggest Learning:

Today's Magic Moment:

Daily Plan

Day at a glance

Time	
6 am	
7 am	
8 am	
9 am	
10 am	
11 am	
12 pm	
1 pm	
2 pm	
3 pm	
4 pm	
5 pm	
6 pm	
7 pm	

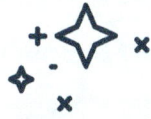

Remember This!

Top Priorities!

Glass of Water Score

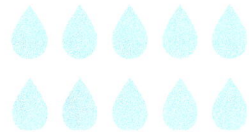

Biggest Learning:

Today's Magic Moment:

Daily Plan

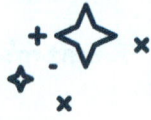

Day at a glance

6 am	
7 am	
8 am	
9 am	
10 am	
11 am	
12 pm	
1 pm	
2 pm	
3 pm	
4 pm	
5 pm	
6 pm	
7 pm	

Top Priorities!

Glass of Water Score

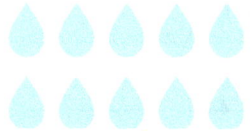

Biggest Learning:

Today's Magic Moment:

Daily Plan

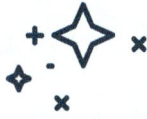

Day at a glance

6 am	
7 am	
8 am	
9 am	
10 am	
11 am	
12 pm	
1 pm	
2 pm	
3 pm	
4 pm	
5 pm	
6 pm	
7 pm	

Remember This!

Top Priorities!

Glass of Water Score

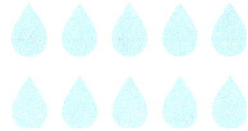

Biggest Learning:

Today's Magic Moment:

Daily Plan

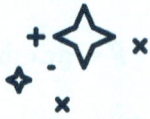

Day at a glance

6 am	
7 am	
8 am	
9 am	
10 am	
11 am	
12 pm	
1 pm	
2 pm	
3 pm	
4 pm	
5 pm	
6 pm	
7 pm	

Remember This!

Top Priorities!

Glass of Water Score

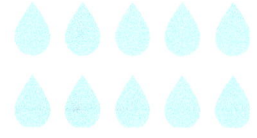

Biggest Learning:

Today's Magic Moment:

Daily Plan

Day at a glance

6 am	
7 am	
8 am	
9 am	
10 am	
11 am	
12 pm	
1 pm	
2 pm	
3 pm	
4 pm	
5 pm	
6 pm	
7 pm	

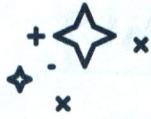

Remember This!

Top Priorities!

Glass of Water Score

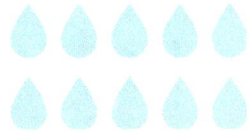

Biggest Learning:

Today's Magic Moment:

Monthly

Focus

Goals	Due By

Results

Tasks

- [ ]
- [ ]
- [ ]
- [ ]
- [ ]
- [ ]

Weekly Snapshot

New Habit
Name It.

Must Do This Week!

Track It.

☐ Mon

☐ Tues

☐ Wed

☐ Thurs

☐ Fri

☐ Sat

☐ Sun

Quote For The Week:

I've learned that people will forget what you said,

people will forget what you did,

but people will never forget how you made them feel.

MAYA ANGELOU

Review It.
How did it go?
What worked?
What didn't?

Daily Plan

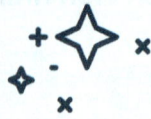

Day at a glance

6 am	
7 am	
8 am	
9 am	
10 am	
11 am	
12 pm	
1 pm	
2 pm	
3 pm	
4 pm	
5 pm	
6 pm	
7 pm	

Remember This!

Top Priorities!

Glass of Water Score

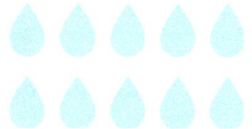

Biggest Learning:

Today's Magic Moment:

Daily Plan

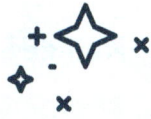

Day at a glance

6 am	
7 am	
8 am	
9 am	
10 am	
11 am	
12 pm	
1 pm	
2 pm	
3 pm	
4 pm	
5 pm	
6 pm	
7 pm	

Remember This!

Top Priorities!

Glass of Water Score

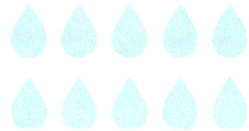

Biggest Learning:

Today's Magic Moment:

Daily
Plan

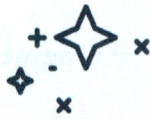

Day at a glance

6 am	
7 am	
8 am	
9 am	
10 am	
11 am	
12 pm	
1 pm	
2 pm	
3 pm	
4 pm	
5 pm	
6 pm	
7 pm	

Top Priorities!

Glass of Water Score

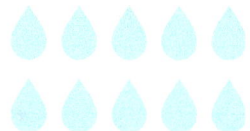

Biggest Learning:

Today's Magic Moment:

Daily Plan

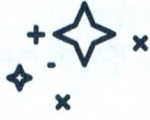

Day at a glance

6 am	
7 am	
8 am	
9 am	
10 am	
11 am	
12 pm	
1 pm	
2 pm	
3 pm	
4 pm	
5 pm	
6 pm	
7 pm	

Remember This!

Top Priorities!

Glass of Water Score

Biggest Learning:

Today's Magic Moment:

Daily Plan

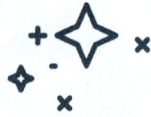

Day at a glance

6 am	
7 am	
8 am	
9 am	
10 am	
11 am	
12 pm	
1 pm	
2 pm	
3 pm	
4 pm	
5 pm	
6 pm	
7 pm	

Remember This!

Top Priorities!

Glass of Water Score

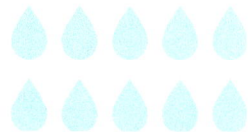

Biggest Learning:

Today's Magic Moment:

Daily Plan

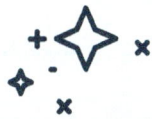

Day at a glance

6 am	
7 am	
8 am	
9 am	
10 am	
11 am	
12 pm	
1 pm	
2 pm	
3 pm	
4 pm	
5 pm	
6 pm	
7 pm	

Remember This!

Top Priorities!

Glass of Water Score

Biggest Learning:

Today's Magic Moment:

Daily Plan

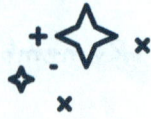

Day at a glance

6 am	
7 am	
8 am	
9 am	
10 am	
11 am	
12 pm	
1 pm	
2 pm	
3 pm	
4 pm	
5 pm	
6 pm	
7 pm	

Remember This!

Top Priorities!

Glass of Water Score

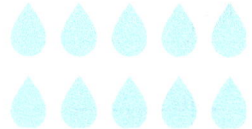

Biggest Learning:

Today's Magic Moment:

Weekly Snapshot

Week Commencing:

New Habit

Name It.

Must Do This Week!

Track It.

- ☐ Mon
- ☐ Tues
- ☐ Wed
- ☐ Thurs
- ☐ Fri
- ☐ Sat
- ☐ Sun

Quote For The Week:

Act as though what you do makes a difference.

It does.

WILLIAM JAMES

Review It.

How did it go?
What worked?
What didn't?

Daily
Plan

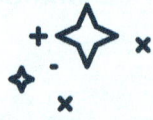

Day at a glance

Remember This!

6 am	
7 am	
8 am	
9 am	
10 am	
11 am	
12 pm	
1 pm	
2 pm	
3 pm	
4 pm	
5 pm	
6 pm	
7 pm	

Top Priorities!

Glass of Water Score

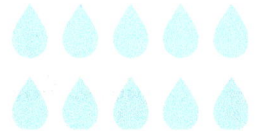

Biggest Learning:

Today's Magic Moment:

Daily Plan

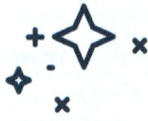

Day at a glance

6 am	
7 am	
8 am	
9 am	
10 am	
11 am	
12 pm	
1 pm	
2 pm	
3 pm	
4 pm	
5 pm	
6 pm	
7 pm	

Remember This!

Top Priorities!

Glass of Water Score

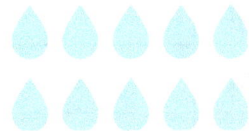

Biggest Learning:

Today's Magic Moment:

Daily Plan

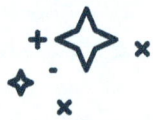

Day at a glance

6 am	
7 am	
8 am	
9 am	
10 am	
11 am	
12 pm	
1 pm	
2 pm	
3 pm	
4 pm	
5 pm	
6 pm	
7 pm	

Remember This!

Top Priorities!

Glass of Water Score

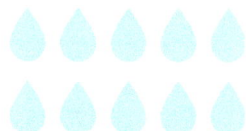

Biggest Learning:

Today's Magic Moment:

Daily Plan

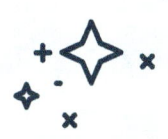

Day at a glance

Remember This!

6 am	
7 am	
8 am	
9 am	
10 am	
11 am	
12 pm	
1 pm	
2 pm	
3 pm	
4 pm	
5 pm	
6 pm	
7 pm	

Top Priorities!

Glass of Water Score

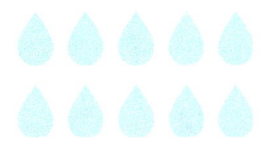

Biggest Learning:

Today's Magic Moment:

Daily Plan

Day at a glance

6 am	
7 am	
8 am	
9 am	
10 am	
11 am	
12 pm	
1 pm	
2 pm	
3 pm	
4 pm	
5 pm	
6 pm	
7 pm	

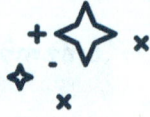

Remember This!

Top Priorities!

Glass of Water Score

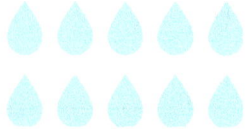

Biggest Learning:

Today's Magic Moment:

Daily Plan

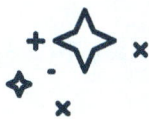

Day at a glance

6 am	
7 am	
8 am	
9 am	
10 am	
11 am	
12 pm	
1 pm	
2 pm	
3 pm	
4 pm	
5 pm	
6 pm	
7 pm	

Remember This!

Top Priorities!

Glass of Water Score

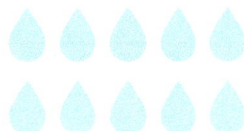

Biggest Learning:

Today's Magic Moment:

Daily Plan

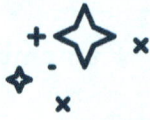

Day at a glance

6 am	
7 am	
8 am	
9 am	
10 am	
11 am	
12 pm	
1 pm	
2 pm	
3 pm	
4 pm	
5 pm	
6 pm	
7 pm	

Remember This!

Top Priorities!

Glass of Water Score

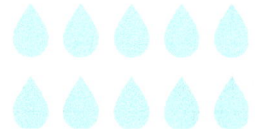

Biggest Learning:

Today's Magic Moment:

Weekly Snapshot

New Habit

Name It.

Must Do This Week!

Track It.

- ☐ Mon
- ☐ Tues
- ☐ Wed
- ☐ Thurs
- ☐ Fri
- ☐ Sat
- ☐ Sun

Quote For The Week:

Don't judge each day by the harvest you reap

but by the seeds that you plant.

ROBERT LOIUS STEVENSON

Review It.
How did it go?
What worked?
What didn't?

Daily Plan

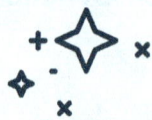

Day at a glance

6 am	
7 am	
8 am	
9 am	
10 am	
11 am	
12 pm	
1 pm	
2 pm	
3 pm	
4 pm	
5 pm	
6 pm	
7 pm	

Remember This!

Top Priorities!

Glass of Water Score

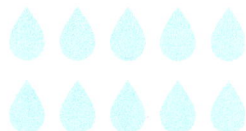

Biggest Learning:

Today's Magic Moment:

Daily Plan

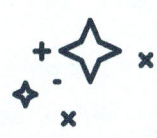

Day at a glance

Time	
6 am	
7 am	
8 am	
9 am	
10 am	
11 am	
12 pm	
1 pm	
2 pm	
3 pm	
4 pm	
5 pm	
6 pm	
7 pm	

Remember This!

Top Priorities!

Glass of Water Score

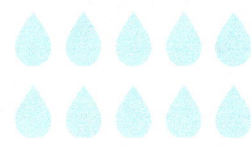

Biggest Learning:

Today's Magic Moment:

Daily
Plan

Day at a glance

6 am	
7 am	
8 am	
9 am	
10 am	
11 am	
12 pm	
1 pm	
2 pm	
3 pm	
4 pm	
5 pm	
6 pm	
7 pm	

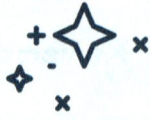

Remember This!

Top Priorities!

Glass of Water Score

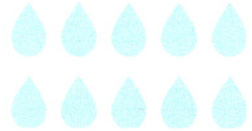

Biggest Learning:

Today's Magic Moment:

Daily
Plan

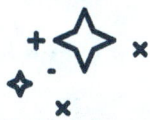

Day at a glance

6 am	
7 am	
8 am	
9 am	
10 am	
11 am	
12 pm	
1 pm	
2 pm	
3 pm	
4 pm	
5 pm	
6 pm	
7 pm	

Top Priorities!

Glass of Water Score

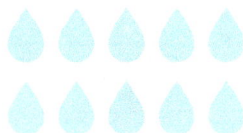

Biggest Learning:

Today's Magic Moment:

Daily
Plan

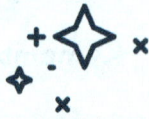

Day at a glance

6 am	
7 am	
8 am	
9 am	
10 am	
11 am	
12 pm	
1 pm	
2 pm	
3 pm	
4 pm	
5 pm	
6 pm	
7 pm	

Top Priorities!

Glass of Water Score

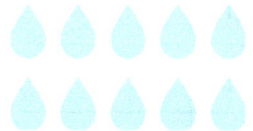

Biggest Learning:

Today's Magic Moment:

Daily Plan

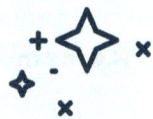

Day at a glance

6 am	
7 am	
8 am	
9 am	
10 am	
11 am	
12 pm	
1 pm	
2 pm	
3 pm	
4 pm	
5 pm	
6 pm	
7 pm	

Remember This!

Top Priorities!

Glass of Water Score

Biggest Learning:

Today's Magic Moment:

Daily Plan

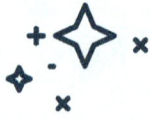

Day at a glance

6 am	
7 am	
8 am	
9 am	
10 am	
11 am	
12 pm	
1 pm	
2 pm	
3 pm	
4 pm	
5 pm	
6 pm	
7 pm	

Top Priorities!

Glass of Water Score

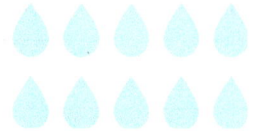

Biggest Learning:

Today's Magic Moment:

Weekly Snapshot

Week Commencing:

New Habit

Name It.

Must Do This Week!

Track It.

- ☐ Mon
- ☐ Tues
- ☐ Wed
- ☐ Thurs
- ☐ Fri
- ☐ Sat
- ☐ Sun

Quote For The Week:

Review It.
How did it go?
What worked?
What didn't?

Daily Plan

Remember This!

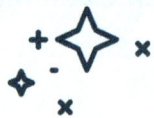

Day at a glance

6 am	
7 am	
8 am	
9 am	
10 am	
11 am	
12 pm	
1 pm	
2 pm	
3 pm	
4 pm	
5 pm	
6 pm	
7 pm	

Top Priorities!

Glass of Water Score

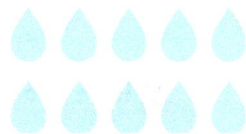

Biggest Learning:

Today's Magic Moment:

Daily
Plan

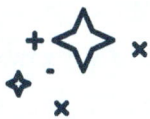

Day at a glance

Remember This!

6 am	
7 am	
8 am	
9 am	
10 am	
11 am	
12 pm	
1 pm	
2 pm	
3 pm	
4 pm	
5 pm	
6 pm	
7 pm	

Top Priorities!

Glass of Water Score

Biggest Learning:

Today's Magic Moment:

Daily Plan

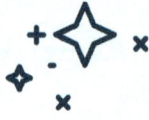

Day at a glance

6 am	
7 am	
8 am	
9 am	
10 am	
11 am	
12 pm	
1 pm	
2 pm	
3 pm	
4 pm	
5 pm	
6 pm	
7 pm	

Remember This!

Top Priorities!

Glass of Water Score

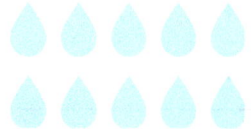

Biggest Learning:

Today's Magic Moment:

Daily
Plan

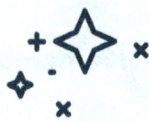

Day at a glance

Remember This!

6 am	
7 am	
8 am	
9 am	
10 am	
11 am	
12 pm	
1 pm	
2 pm	
3 pm	
4 pm	
5 pm	
6 pm	
7 pm	

Top Priorities!

Glass of Water Score

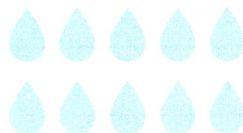

💧💧💧💧💧
💧💧💧💧💧

Biggest Learning:

Today's Magic Moment:

Daily Plan

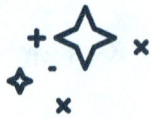

Day at a glance

6 am	
7 am	
8 am	
9 am	
10 am	
11 am	
12 pm	
1 pm	
2 pm	
3 pm	
4 pm	
5 pm	
6 pm	
7 pm	

Remember This!

Top Priorities!

Glass of Water Score

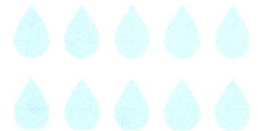

Biggest Learning:

Today's Magic Moment:

Daily Plan

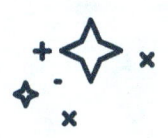

Day at a glance

Time	
6 am	
7 am	
8 am	
9 am	
10 am	
11 am	
12 pm	
1 pm	
2 pm	
3 pm	
4 pm	
5 pm	
6 pm	
7 pm	

Remember This!

Top Priorities!

Glass of Water Score

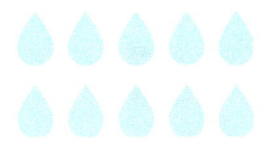

Biggest Learning:

Today's Magic Moment:

Daily Plan

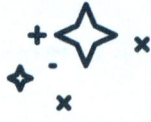

Day at a glance

Time	
6 am	
7 am	
8 am	
9 am	
10 am	
11 am	
12 pm	
1 pm	
2 pm	
3 pm	
4 pm	
5 pm	
6 pm	
7 pm	

Remember This!

Top Priorities!

Glass of Water Score

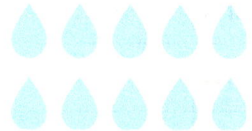

Biggest Learning:

Today's Magic Moment:

Weekly
Snapshot

New Habit

Name It.

Must Do This Week!

Track It.

- ☐ Mon
- ☐ Tues
- ☐ Wed
- ☐ Thurs
- ☐ Fri
- ☐ Sat
- ☐ Sun

Quote For The Week:

Our greatest weakness lies in giving up.

The most certain way to succeed is always to try just one more time.

THOMAS A. EDISON

Review It.
How did it go?
What worked?
What didn't?

Daily
Plan

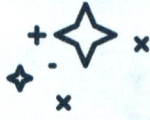

Day at a glance

Remember This!

6 am	
7 am	
8 am	
9 am	
10 am	
11 am	
12 pm	
1 pm	
2 pm	
3 pm	
4 pm	
5 pm	
6 pm	
7 pm	

Top Priorities!

Glass of Water Score

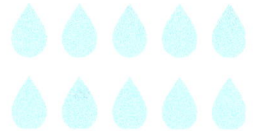

Biggest Learning:

Today's Magic Moment:

Daily
Plan

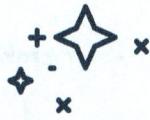

Day at a glance

6 am	
7 am	
8 am	
9 am	
10 am	
11 am	
12 pm	
1 pm	
2 pm	
3 pm	
4 pm	
5 pm	
6 pm	
7 pm	

Remember This!

Top Priorities!

Glass of Water Score

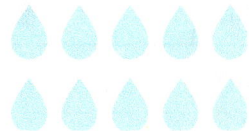

Biggest Learning:

Today's Magic Moment:

Daily
Plan

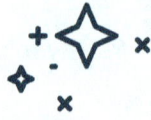

Day at a glance

6 am	
7 am	
8 am	
9 am	
10 am	
11 am	
12 pm	
1 pm	
2 pm	
3 pm	
4 pm	
5 pm	
6 pm	
7 pm	

Top Priorities!

Glass of Water Score

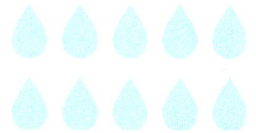

Biggest Learning:

Today's Magic Moment:

Daily Plan

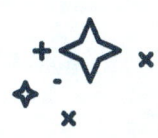

Day at a glance

6 am	
7 am	
8 am	
9 am	
10 am	
11 am	
12 pm	
1 pm	
2 pm	
3 pm	
4 pm	
5 pm	
6 pm	
7 pm	

Remember This!

Top Priorities!

Glass of Water Score

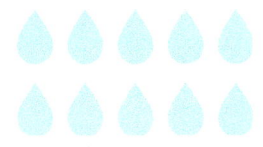

💧 💧 💧 💧 💧

💧 💧 💧 💧 💧

Biggest Learning:

Today's Magic Moment:

Daily Plan

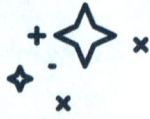

Day at a glance

6 am	
7 am	
8 am	
9 am	
10 am	
11 am	
12 pm	
1 pm	
2 pm	
3 pm	
4 pm	
5 pm	
6 pm	
7 pm	

Remember This!

Top Priorities!

Glass of Water Score

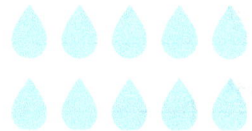

Biggest Learning:

Today's Magic Moment:

Daily
Plan

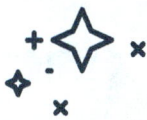

Day at a glance

6 am	
7 am	
8 am	
9 am	
10 am	
11 am	
12 pm	
1 pm	
2 pm	
3 pm	
4 pm	
5 pm	
6 pm	
7 pm	

Remember This!

Top Priorities!

Glass of Water Score

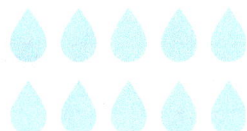

Biggest Learning:

Today's Magic Moment:

Daily
Plan

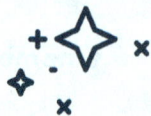

Day at a glance

6 am	
7 am	
8 am	
9 am	
10 am	
11 am	
12 pm	
1 pm	
2 pm	
3 pm	
4 pm	
5 pm	
6 pm	
7 pm	

Top Priorities!

Glass of Water Score

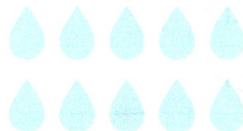

Biggest Learning:

Today's Magic Moment:

Monthly
Focus

Goals	Due By

Tasks

- [ ]
- [ ]
- [ ]
- [ ]
- [ ]
- [ ]

Results

Weekly Snapshot

Week Commencing:

Must Do This Week!

New Habit
Name It.

Track It.

- ☐ Mon
- ☐ Tues
- ☐ Wed
- ☐ Thurs
- ☐ Fri
- ☐ Sat
- ☐ Sun

Quote For The Week:

You can't go back and change the beginning,

but you can start where you are and change the ending.

C. S. LEWIS

Review It.
How did it go?
What worked?
What didn't?

Daily Plan

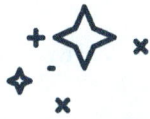

Day at a glance

6 am	
7 am	
8 am	
9 am	
10 am	
11 am	
12 pm	
1 pm	
2 pm	
3 pm	
4 pm	
5 pm	
6 pm	
7 pm	

Remember This!

Top Priorities!

Glass of Water Score

Biggest Learning:

Today's Magic Moment:

Daily Plan

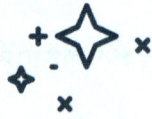

Day at a glance

Time	
6 am	
7 am	
8 am	
9 am	
10 am	
11 am	
12 pm	
1 pm	
2 pm	
3 pm	
4 pm	
5 pm	
6 pm	
7 pm	

Remember This!

Top Priorities!

Glass of Water Score

Biggest Learning:

Today's Magic Moment:

Daily
Plan

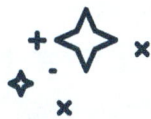

Day at a glance

6 am	
7 am	
8 am	
9 am	
10 am	
11 am	
12 pm	
1 pm	
2 pm	
3 pm	
4 pm	
5 pm	
6 pm	
7 pm	

Remember This!

Top Priorities!

Glass of Water Score

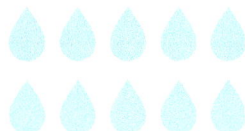

Biggest Learning:

Today's Magic Moment:

Daily Plan

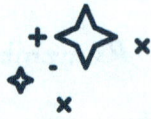

Day at a glance

6 am	
7 am	
8 am	
9 am	
10 am	
11 am	
12 pm	
1 pm	
2 pm	
3 pm	
4 pm	
5 pm	
6 pm	
7 pm	

Remember This!

Top Priorities!

Glass of Water Score

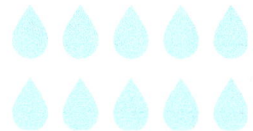

Biggest Learning:

Today's Magic Moment:

Daily Plan

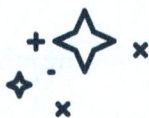

Day at a glance

6 am	
7 am	
8 am	
9 am	
10 am	
11 am	
12 pm	
1 pm	
2 pm	
3 pm	
4 pm	
5 pm	
6 pm	
7 pm	

Remember This!

Top Priorities!

Glass of Water Score

Biggest Learning:

Today's Magic Moment:

Daily
Plan

Day at a glance

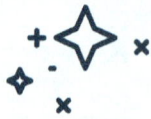

Remember This!

6 am	
7 am	
8 am	
9 am	
10 am	
11 am	
12 pm	
1 pm	
2 pm	
3 pm	
4 pm	
5 pm	
6 pm	
7 pm	

Top Priorities!

Glass of Water Score

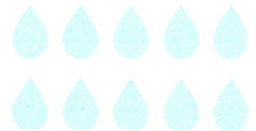

Biggest Learning:

Today's Magic Moment:

Daily Plan

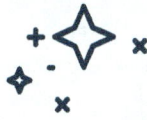

Day at a glance

6 am	
7 am	
8 am	
9 am	
10 am	
11 am	
12 pm	
1 pm	
2 pm	
3 pm	
4 pm	
5 pm	
6 pm	
7 pm	

Remember This!

Top Priorities!

Glass of Water Score

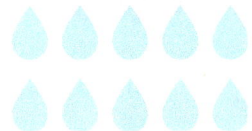

Biggest Learning:

Today's Magic Moment:

Weekly Snapshot

Week Commencing:

New Habit
Name It.

Must Do This Week!

Track It.

- ☐ Mon
- ☐ Tues
- ☐ Wed
- ☐ Thurs
- ☐ Fri
- ☐ Sat
- ☐ Sun

Quote For The Week:

Review It.
How did it go?
What worked?
What didn't?

Daily
Plan

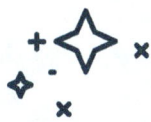

Day at a glance

6 am	
7 am	
8 am	
9 am	
10 am	
11 am	
12 pm	
1 pm	
2 pm	
3 pm	
4 pm	
5 pm	
6 pm	
7 pm	

Remember This!

Top Priorities!

Glass of Water Score

Biggest Learning:

Today's Magic Moment:

Daily
Plan

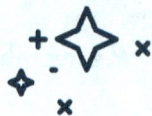

Day at a glance

Time	
6 am	
7 am	
8 am	
9 am	
10 am	
11 am	
12 pm	
1 pm	
2 pm	
3 pm	
4 pm	
5 pm	
6 pm	
7 pm	

Remember This!

Top Priorities!

Glass of Water Score

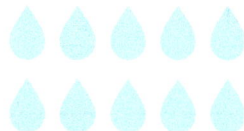

Biggest Learning:

Today's Magic Moment:

Daily Plan

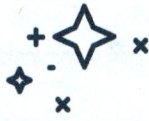

Day at a glance

6 am	
7 am	
8 am	
9 am	
10 am	
11 am	
12 pm	
1 pm	
2 pm	
3 pm	
4 pm	
5 pm	
6 pm	
7 pm	

Remember This!

Top Priorities!

Glass of Water Score

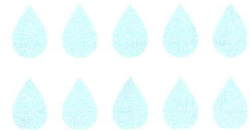

Biggest Learning:

Today's Magic Moment:

Daily

Plan

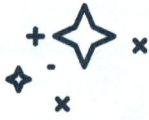

Day at a glance

6 am	
7 am	
8 am	
9 am	
10 am	
11 am	
12 pm	
1 pm	
2 pm	
3 pm	
4 pm	
5 pm	
6 pm	
7 pm	

Top Priorities!

Glass of Water Score

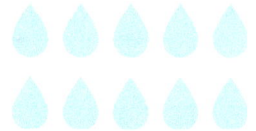

Biggest Learning:

Today's Magic Moment:

Daily Plan

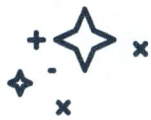

Day at a glance

6 am	
7 am	
8 am	
9 am	
10 am	
11 am	
12 pm	
1 pm	
2 pm	
3 pm	
4 pm	
5 pm	
6 pm	
7 pm	

Remember This!

Top Priorities!

Glass of Water Score

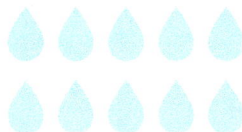

Biggest Learning:

Today's Magic Moment:

Daily
Plan

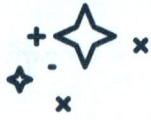

Day at a glance

6 am	
7 am	
8 am	
9 am	
10 am	
11 am	
12 pm	
1 pm	
2 pm	
3 pm	
4 pm	
5 pm	
6 pm	
7 pm	

Top Priorities!

Glass of Water Score

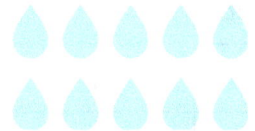

Biggest Learning:

Today's Magic Moment:

Daily Plan

Day at a glance

6 am	
7 am	
8 am	
9 am	
10 am	
11 am	
12 pm	
1 pm	
2 pm	
3 pm	
4 pm	
5 pm	
6 pm	
7 pm	

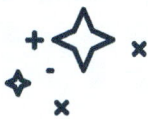

Remember This!

Top Priorities!

Glass of Water Score

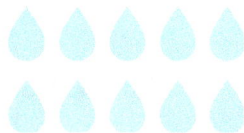

Biggest Learning:

Today's Magic Moment:

Weekly Snapshot

Week Commencing:

New Habit

Name It.

Must Do This Week!

Track It.

- ☐ Mon
- ☐ Tues
- ☐ Wed
- ☐ Thurs
- ☐ Fri
- ☐ Sat
- ☐ Sun

Quote For The Week:

The only man who never makes mistakes

is the man who never does anything.

THEODORE ROOSEVELT

Review It.
How did it go?
What worked?
What didn't?

Daily Plan

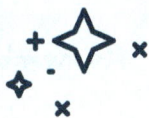

Day at a glance

Time	
6 am	
7 am	
8 am	
9 am	
10 am	
11 am	
12 pm	
1 pm	
2 pm	
3 pm	
4 pm	
5 pm	
6 pm	
7 pm	

Remember This!

Top Priorities!

Glass of Water Score

Biggest Learning:

Today's Magic Moment:

Daily
Plan

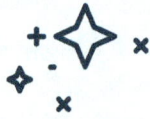

Day at a glance

6 am	
7 am	
8 am	
9 am	
10 am	
11 am	
12 pm	
1 pm	
2 pm	
3 pm	
4 pm	
5 pm	
6 pm	
7 pm	

Remember This!

Top Priorities!

Glass of Water Score

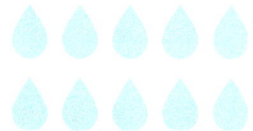

Biggest Learning:

Today's Magic Moment:

Daily Plan

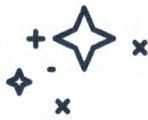

Day at a glance

6 am	
7 am	
8 am	
9 am	
10 am	
11 am	
12 pm	
1 pm	
2 pm	
3 pm	
4 pm	
5 pm	
6 pm	
7 pm	

Remember This!

Top Priorities!

Glass of Water Score

Biggest Learning:

Today's Magic Moment:

Daily Plan

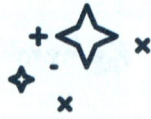

Day at a glance

6 am	
7 am	
8 am	
9 am	
10 am	
11 am	
12 pm	
1 pm	
2 pm	
3 pm	
4 pm	
5 pm	
6 pm	
7 pm	

Remember This!

Top Priorities!

Glass of Water Score

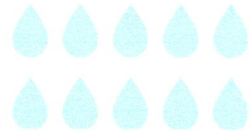

Biggest Learning:

Today's Magic Moment:

Daily
Plan

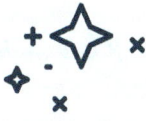

Day at a glance

6 am	
7 am	
8 am	
9 am	
10 am	
11 am	
12 pm	
1 pm	
2 pm	
3 pm	
4 pm	
5 pm	
6 pm	
7 pm	

Remember This!

Top Priorities!

Glass of Water Score

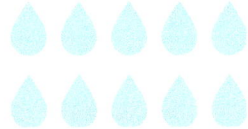

Biggest Learning:

Today's Magic Moment:

Daily Plan

Day at a glance

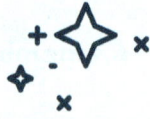

Remember This!

6 am	
7 am	
8 am	
9 am	
10 am	
11 am	
12 pm	
1 pm	
2 pm	
3 pm	
4 pm	
5 pm	
6 pm	
7 pm	

Top Priorities!

Glass of Water Score

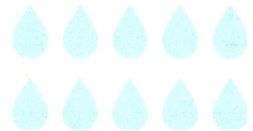

Biggest Learning:

Today's Magic Moment:

Daily

Plan

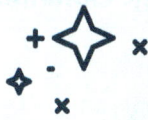

Day at a glance

6 am	
7 am	
8 am	
9 am	
10 am	
11 am	
12 pm	
1 pm	
2 pm	
3 pm	
4 pm	
5 pm	
6 pm	
7 pm	

Remember This!

Top Priorities!

Glass of Water Score

Biggest Learning:

Today's Magic Moment:

Weekly
Snapshot

Week Commencing:

New Habit
Name It.

Must Do This Week!

Track It.

- ☐ Mon
- ☐ Tues
- ☐ Wed
- ☐ Thurs
- ☐ Fri
- ☐ Sat
- ☐ Sun

Quote For The Week:

If opportunity doesn't knock,

build a door.

MILTON BERLE

Review It.
How did it go?
What worked?
What didn't?

Daily Plan

Remember This! ☝️

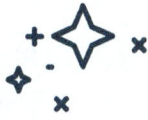

Day at a glance

Time	
6 am	
7 am	
8 am	
9 am	
10 am	
11 am	
12 pm	
1 pm	
2 pm	
3 pm	
4 pm	
5 pm	
6 pm	
7 pm	

Top Priorities!

Glass of Water Score

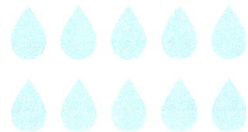

💧💧💧💧💧
💧💧💧💧💧

Biggest Learning:

Today's Magic Moment:

Daily Plan

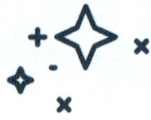

Day at a glance

6 am	
7 am	
8 am	
9 am	
10 am	
11 am	
12 pm	
1 pm	
2 pm	
3 pm	
4 pm	
5 pm	
6 pm	
7 pm	

Remember This!

Top Priorities!

Glass of Water Score

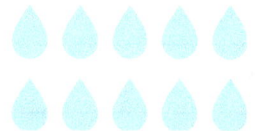

Biggest Learning:

Today's Magic Moment:

Daily
Plan

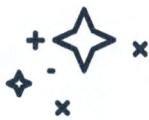

Day at a glance

Remember This!

6 am	
7 am	
8 am	
9 am	
10 am	
11 am	
12 pm	
1 pm	
2 pm	
3 pm	
4 pm	
5 pm	
6 pm	
7 pm	

Top Priorities!

Glass of Water Score

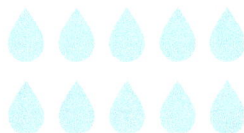

Biggest Learning:

Today's Magic Moment:

Daily
Plan

Day at a glance

6 am	
7 am	
8 am	
9 am	
10 am	
11 am	
12 pm	
1 pm	
2 pm	
3 pm	
4 pm	
5 pm	
6 pm	
7 pm	

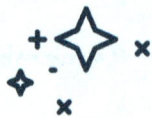

Remember This!

Top Priorities!

Glass of Water Score

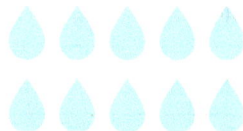

Biggest Learning:

Today's Magic Moment:

Daily Plan

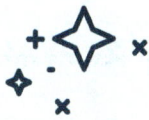

Day at a glance

6 am	
7 am	
8 am	
9 am	
10 am	
11 am	
12 pm	
1 pm	
2 pm	
3 pm	
4 pm	
5 pm	
6 pm	
7 pm	

Remember This!

Top Priorities!

Glass of Water Score

Biggest Learning:

Today's Magic Moment:

Daily Plan

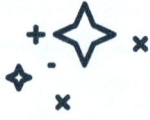

Day at a glance

Remember This!

6 am	
7 am	
8 am	
9 am	
10 am	
11 am	
12 pm	
1 pm	
2 pm	
3 pm	
4 pm	
5 pm	
6 pm	
7 pm	

Top Priorities!

Glass of Water Score

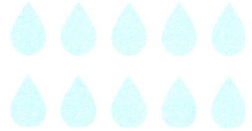

Biggest Learning:

Today's Magic Moment:

Daily Plan

Day at a glance

Time	
6 am	
7 am	
8 am	
9 am	
10 am	
11 am	
12 pm	
1 pm	
2 pm	
3 pm	
4 pm	
5 pm	
6 pm	
7 pm	

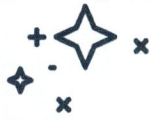

Remember This!

Top Priorities!

Glass of Water Score

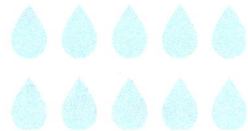

Biggest Learning:

Today's Magic Moment:

Weekly Snapshot

Week Commencing:

New Habit
Name It.

Must Do This Week!

Track It.

- ☐ Mon
- ☐ Tues
- ☐ Wed
- ☐ Thurs
- ☐ Fri
- ☐ Sat
- ☐ Sun

Quote For The Week:

Quality is never an accident;

it is always the result

of intelligent effort.

JOHN RUSKIN

Review It.
How did it go?
What worked?
What didn't?

Daily
Plan

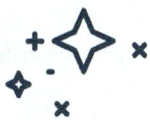

Day at a glance

6 am	
7 am	
8 am	
9 am	
10 am	
11 am	
12 pm	
1 pm	
2 pm	
3 pm	
4 pm	
5 pm	
6 pm	
7 pm	

Remember This!

Top Priorities!

Glass of Water Score

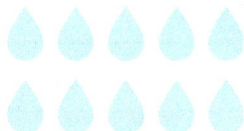

Biggest Learning:

Today's Magic Moment:

Daily Plan

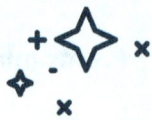

Day at a glance

6 am	
7 am	
8 am	
9 am	
10 am	
11 am	
12 pm	
1 pm	
2 pm	
3 pm	
4 pm	
5 pm	
6 pm	
7 pm	

Remember This!

Top Priorities!

Glass of Water Score

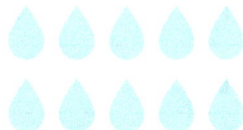

Biggest Learning:

Today's Magic Moment:

Daily
Plan

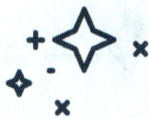

Day at a glance

6 am	
7 am	
8 am	
9 am	
10 am	
11 am	
12 pm	
1 pm	
2 pm	
3 pm	
4 pm	
5 pm	
6 pm	
7 pm	

Remember This!

Top Priorities!

Glass of Water Score

Biggest Learning:

Today's Magic Moment:

Daily Plan

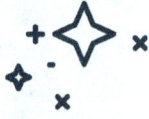

Day at a glance

6 am	
7 am	
8 am	
9 am	
10 am	
11 am	
12 pm	
1 pm	
2 pm	
3 pm	
4 pm	
5 pm	
6 pm	
7 pm	

Remember This!

Top Priorities!

Glass of Water Score

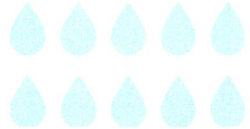

Biggest Learning:

Today's Magic Moment:

Daily Plan

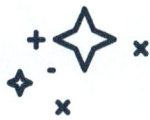

Day at a glance

6 am	
7 am	
8 am	
9 am	
10 am	
11 am	
12 pm	
1 pm	
2 pm	
3 pm	
4 pm	
5 pm	
6 pm	
7 pm	

Remember This!

Top Priorities!

Glass of Water Score

Biggest Learning:

Today's Magic Moment:

Daily
Plan

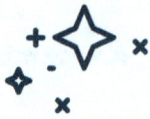

Day at a glance

Remember This!

6 am	
7 am	
8 am	
9 am	
10 am	
11 am	
12 pm	
1 pm	
2 pm	
3 pm	
4 pm	
5 pm	
6 pm	
7 pm	

Top Priorities!

Glass of Water Score

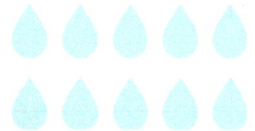

Biggest Learning:

Today's Magic Moment:

Daily Plan

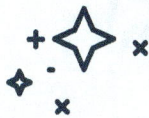

Day at a glance

Time	
6 am	
7 am	
8 am	
9 am	
10 am	
11 am	
12 pm	
1 pm	
2 pm	
3 pm	
4 pm	
5 pm	
6 pm	
7 pm	

Biggest Learning:

Remember This!

Top Priorities!

Glass of Water Score

Today's Magic Moment:

Monthly

Focus

Goals	Due By

Results

Tasks

- [ ]
- [ ]
- [ ]
- [ ]
- [ ]
- [ ]

Weekly Snapshot

Week Commencing:

Must Do This Week!

New Habit
Name It.

Track It.

- ☐ Mon
- ☐ Tues
- ☐ Wed
- ☐ Thurs
- ☐ Fri
- ☐ Sat
- ☐ Sun

Quote For The Week:

Quality means doing it right
when no one is looking.

HENRY FORD

Review It.
How did it go?
What worked?
What didn't?

Daily
Plan

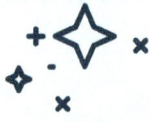

Day at a glance

6 am	
7 am	
8 am	
9 am	
10 am	
11 am	
12 pm	
1 pm	
2 pm	
3 pm	
4 pm	
5 pm	
6 pm	
7 pm	

Top Priorities!

Glass of Water Score

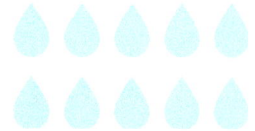

Biggest Learning:

Today's Magic Moment:

Daily Plan

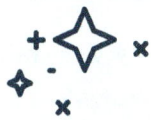

Day at a glance

Remember This!

Time	
6 am	
7 am	
8 am	
9 am	
10 am	
11 am	
12 pm	
1 pm	
2 pm	
3 pm	
4 pm	
5 pm	
6 pm	
7 pm	

Top Priorities!

Glass of Water Score

Biggest Learning:

Today's Magic Moment:

Daily Plan

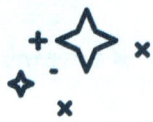

Day at a glance

6 am	
7 am	
8 am	
9 am	
10 am	
11 am	
12 pm	
1 pm	
2 pm	
3 pm	
4 pm	
5 pm	
6 pm	
7 pm	

Remember This!

Top Priorities!

Glass of Water Score

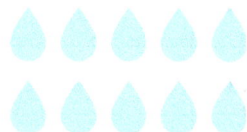

Biggest Learning:

Today's Magic Moment:

Daily
Plan

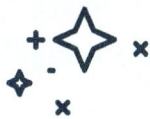

Day at a glance

6 am	
7 am	
8 am	
9 am	
10 am	
11 am	
12 pm	
1 pm	
2 pm	
3 pm	
4 pm	
5 pm	
6 pm	
7 pm	

Remember This!

Top Priorities!

Glass of Water Score

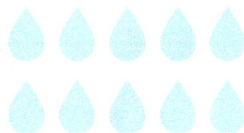

Biggest Learning:

Today's Magic Moment:

Daily Plan

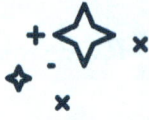

Day at a glance

6 am	
7 am	
8 am	
9 am	
10 am	
11 am	
12 pm	
1 pm	
2 pm	
3 pm	
4 pm	
5 pm	
6 pm	
7 pm	

Remember This!

Top Priorities!

Glass of Water Score

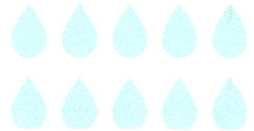

Biggest Learning:

Today's Magic Moment:

Daily

Plan

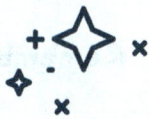

Day at a glance

6 am	
7 am	
8 am	
9 am	
10 am	
11 am	
12 pm	
1 pm	
2 pm	
3 pm	
4 pm	
5 pm	
6 pm	
7 pm	

Remember This!

Top Priorities!

Glass of Water Score

Biggest Learning:

Today's Magic Moment:

Daily Plan

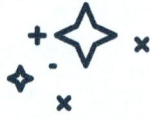

Day at a glance

6 am	
7 am	
8 am	
9 am	
10 am	
11 am	
12 pm	
1 pm	
2 pm	
3 pm	
4 pm	
5 pm	
6 pm	
7 pm	

Remember This!

Top Priorities!

Glass of Water Score

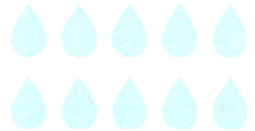

Biggest Learning:

Today's Magic Moment:

Weekly
Snapshot

Week Commencing:

New Habit

Name It.

Must Do This Week!

Track It.

☐ Mon

☐ Tues

☐ Wed

☐ Thurs

☐ Fri

☐ Sat

☐ Sun

Quote For The Week:

Review It.
How did it go?
What worked?
What didn't?

Daily Plan

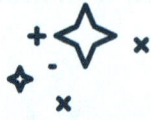

Day at a glance

6 am	
7 am	
8 am	
9 am	
10 am	
11 am	
12 pm	
1 pm	
2 pm	
3 pm	
4 pm	
5 pm	
6 pm	
7 pm	

Remember This!

Top Priorities!

Glass of Water Score

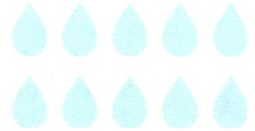

Biggest Learning:

Today's Magic Moment:

Daily
Plan

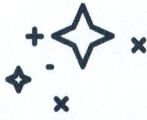

Day at a glance

6 am	
7 am	
8 am	
9 am	
10 am	
11 am	
12 pm	
1 pm	
2 pm	
3 pm	
4 pm	
5 pm	
6 pm	
7 pm	

Remember This!

Top Priorities!

Glass of Water Score

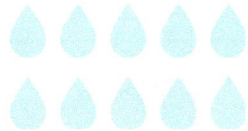

Biggest Learning:

Today's Magic Moment:

Daily Plan

Day at a glance

6 am	
7 am	
8 am	
9 am	
10 am	
11 am	
12 pm	
1 pm	
2 pm	
3 pm	
4 pm	
5 pm	
6 pm	
7 pm	

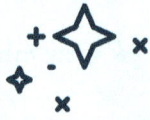

Remember This!

Top Priorities!

Glass of Water Score

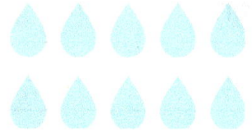

Biggest Learning:

Today's Magic Moment:

Daily
Plan

Remember This!

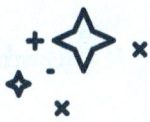

Day at a glance

6 am	
7 am	
8 am	
9 am	
10 am	
11 am	
12 pm	
1 pm	
2 pm	
3 pm	
4 pm	
5 pm	
6 pm	
7 pm	

Top Priorities!

Glass of Water Score

Biggest Learning:

Today's Magic Moment:

Daily Plan

Remember This!

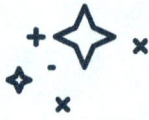

Day at a glance

6 am	
7 am	
8 am	
9 am	
10 am	
11 am	
12 pm	
1 pm	
2 pm	
3 pm	
4 pm	
5 pm	
6 pm	
7 pm	

Top Priorities!

Glass of Water Score

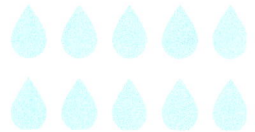

Biggest Learning:

Today's Magic Moment:

Daily

Plan

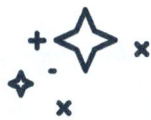

Day at a glance

6 am	
7 am	
8 am	
9 am	
10 am	
11 am	
12 pm	
1 pm	
2 pm	
3 pm	
4 pm	
5 pm	
6 pm	
7 pm	

Remember This!

Top Priorities!

Glass of Water Score

Biggest Learning:

Today's Magic Moment:

Daily Plan

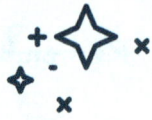

Day at a glance

6 am	
7 am	
8 am	
9 am	
10 am	
11 am	
12 pm	
1 pm	
2 pm	
3 pm	
4 pm	
5 pm	
6 pm	
7 pm	

Top Priorities!

Glass of Water Score

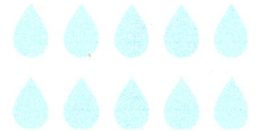

Biggest Learning:

Today's Magic Moment:

Weekly Snapshot

New Habit

Name It.

Must Do This Week!

Track It.

- ☐ Mon
- ☐ Tues
- ☐ Wed
- ☐ Thurs
- ☐ Fri
- ☐ Sat
- ☐ Sun

Quote For The Week:

Real magic in relationships
means an absence of
judgement of others.

WAYNE DYER

Review It.
How did it go?
What worked?
What didn't?

Daily Plan

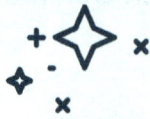

Day at a glance

6 am	
7 am	
8 am	
9 am	
10 am	
11 am	
12 pm	
1 pm	
2 pm	
3 pm	
4 pm	
5 pm	
6 pm	
7 pm	

Remember This!

Top Priorities!

Glass of Water Score

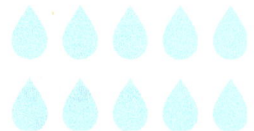

Biggest Learning:

Today's Magic Moment:

Daily
Plan

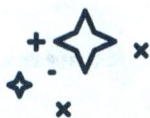

Day at a glance

6 am	
7 am	
8 am	
9 am	
10 am	
11 am	
12 pm	
1 pm	
2 pm	
3 pm	
4 pm	
5 pm	
6 pm	
7 pm	

Remember This!

Top Priorities!

Glass of Water Score

Biggest Learning:

Today's Magic Moment:

Daily Plan

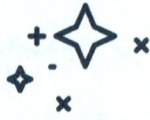

Day at a glance

Remember This!

6 am	
7 am	
8 am	
9 am	
10 am	
11 am	
12 pm	
1 pm	
2 pm	
3 pm	
4 pm	
5 pm	
6 pm	
7 pm	

Top Priorities!

Glass of Water Score

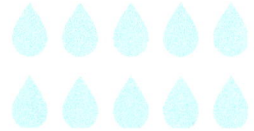

Biggest Learning:

Today's Magic Moment:

Daily

Plan

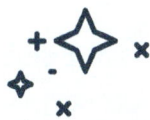

Day at a glance

6 am	
7 am	
8 am	
9 am	
10 am	
11 am	
12 pm	
1 pm	
2 pm	
3 pm	
4 pm	
5 pm	
6 pm	
7 pm	

Remember This!

Top Priorities!

Glass of Water Score

Biggest Learning:

Today's Magic Moment:

Daily Plan

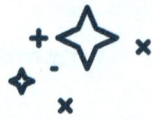

Day at a glance

6 am	
7 am	
8 am	
9 am	
10 am	
11 am	
12 pm	
1 pm	
2 pm	
3 pm	
4 pm	
5 pm	
6 pm	
7 pm	

Remember This!

Top Priorities!

Glass of Water Score

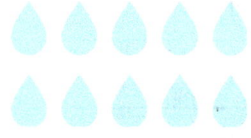

Biggest Learning:

Today's Magic Moment:

Daily Plan

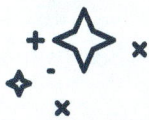

Day at a glance

Time	
6 am	
7 am	
8 am	
9 am	
10 am	
11 am	
12 pm	
1 pm	
2 pm	
3 pm	
4 pm	
5 pm	
6 pm	
7 pm	

Remember This!

Top Priorities!

Glass of Water Score

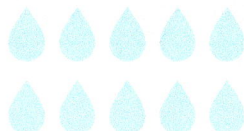

Biggest Learning:

Today's Magic Moment:

Daily Plan

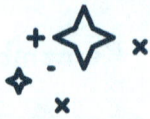

Day at a glance

Time	
6 am	
7 am	
8 am	
9 am	
10 am	
11 am	
12 pm	
1 pm	
2 pm	
3 pm	
4 pm	
5 pm	
6 pm	
7 pm	

Top Priorities!

Glass of Water Score

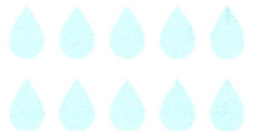

Biggest Learning:

Today's Magic Moment:

Weekly Snapshot

Week Commencing:

New Habit

Name It.

Track It.

- ☐ Mon
- ☐ Tues
- ☐ Wed
- ☐ Thurs
- ☐ Fri
- ☐ Sat
- ☐ Sun

Must Do This Week!

_____

_____

_____

_____

_____

_____

_____

Review It.
How did it go?
What worked?
What didn't?

Quote For The Week:

IN THE END...

We only regret the chances
we didn't take,

the relationships we were
afraid to have,

and the decisions we waited
too long to make.

LEWIS CARROLL

Daily
Plan

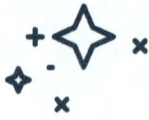

Day at a glance

6 am	
7 am	
8 am	
9 am	
10 am	
11 am	
12 pm	
1 pm	
2 pm	
3 pm	
4 pm	
5 pm	
6 pm	
7 pm	

Top Priorities!

Glass of Water Score

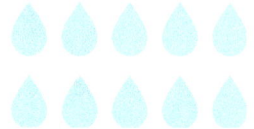

Biggest Learning:

Today's Magic Moment:

Daily Plan

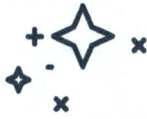

Day at a glance

6 am	
7 am	
8 am	
9 am	
10 am	
11 am	
12 pm	
1 pm	
2 pm	
3 pm	
4 pm	
5 pm	
6 pm	
7 pm	

Remember This!

Top Priorities!

Glass of Water Score

Biggest Learning:

Today's Magic Moment:

Daily Plan

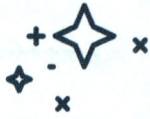

Day at a glance

6 am	
7 am	
8 am	
9 am	
10 am	
11 am	
12 pm	
1 pm	
2 pm	
3 pm	
4 pm	
5 pm	
6 pm	
7 pm	

Top Priorities!

Glass of Water Score

Biggest Learning:

Today's Magic Moment:

Daily Plan

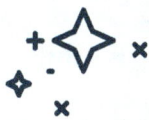

Day at a glance

Remember This!

6 am	
7 am	
8 am	
9 am	
10 am	
11 am	
12 pm	
1 pm	
2 pm	
3 pm	
4 pm	
5 pm	
6 pm	
7 pm	

Top Priorities!

Glass of Water Score

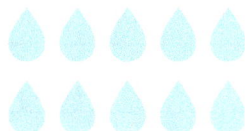

Biggest Learning:

Today's Magic Moment:

Daily Plan

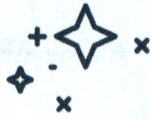

Day at a glance

Remember This!

6 am	
7 am	
8 am	
9 am	
10 am	
11 am	
12 pm	
1 pm	
2 pm	
3 pm	
4 pm	
5 pm	
6 pm	
7 pm	

Top Priorities!

Glass of Water Score

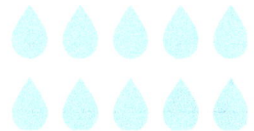

Biggest Learning:

Today's Magic Moment:

Daily Plan

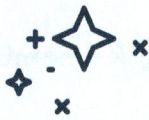

Day at a glance

6 am	
7 am	
8 am	
9 am	
10 am	
11 am	
12 pm	
1 pm	
2 pm	
3 pm	
4 pm	
5 pm	
6 pm	
7 pm	

Remember This!

Top Priorities!

Glass of Water Score

Biggest Learning:

Today's Magic Moment:

Daily Plan

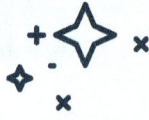

Day at a glance

Time	
6 am	
7 am	
8 am	
9 am	
10 am	
11 am	
12 pm	
1 pm	
2 pm	
3 pm	
4 pm	
5 pm	
6 pm	
7 pm	

Remember This!

Top Priorities!

Glass of Water Score

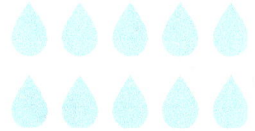

Biggest Learning:

Today's Magic Moment:

Weekly Snapshot

New Habit

Name It.

Must Do This Week!

Track It.

- ☐ Mon
- ☐ Tues
- ☐ Wed
- ☐ Thurs
- ☐ Fri
- ☐ Sat
- ☐ Sun

Quote For The Week:

Appreciation can make a day,
even change a life.
Your willingness to put it into
words is all that is necessary.

MARGARET COUSINS

Review It.

How did it go?
What worked?
What didn't?

Daily Plan

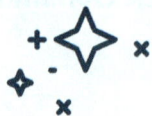

Day at a glance

6 am	
7 am	
8 am	
9 am	
10 am	
11 am	
12 pm	
1 pm	
2 pm	
3 pm	
4 pm	
5 pm	
6 pm	
7 pm	

Remember This!

Top Priorities!

Glass of Water Score

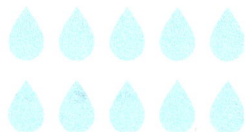

Biggest Learning:

Today's Magic Moment:

Daily
Plan

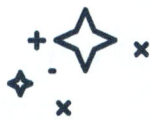

Day at a glance

6 am	
7 am	
8 am	
9 am	
10 am	
11 am	
12 pm	
1 pm	
2 pm	
3 pm	
4 pm	
5 pm	
6 pm	
7 pm	

Top Priorities!

Glass of Water Score

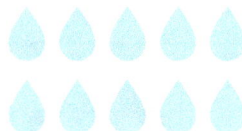

Biggest Learning:

Today's Magic Moment:

Daily Plan

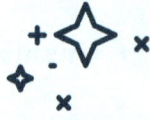

Day at a glance

6 am	
7 am	
8 am	
9 am	
10 am	
11 am	
12 pm	
1 pm	
2 pm	
3 pm	
4 pm	
5 pm	
6 pm	
7 pm	

Remember This!

Top Priorities!

Glass of Water Score

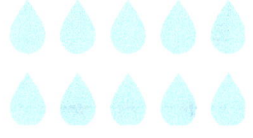

Biggest Learning:

Today's Magic Moment:

Daily
Plan

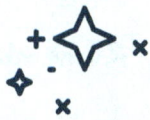

Day at a glance

6 am	
7 am	
8 am	
9 am	
10 am	
11 am	
12 pm	
1 pm	
2 pm	
3 pm	
4 pm	
5 pm	
6 pm	
7 pm	

Remember This!

Top Priorities!

Glass of Water Score

Biggest Learning:

Today's Magic Moment:

Daily Plan

Remember This!

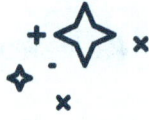

Day at a glance

Time	
6 am	
7 am	
8 am	
9 am	
10 am	
11 am	
12 pm	
1 pm	
2 pm	
3 pm	
4 pm	
5 pm	
6 pm	
7 pm	

Top Priorities!

Glass of Water Score

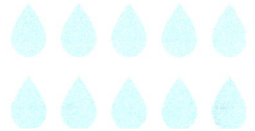

Biggest Learning:

Today's Magic Moment:

Daily
Plan

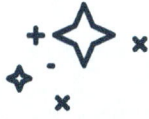

Day at a glance

6 am	
7 am	
8 am	
9 am	
10 am	
11 am	
12 pm	
1 pm	
2 pm	
3 pm	
4 pm	
5 pm	
6 pm	
7 pm	

Top Priorities!

Glass of Water Score

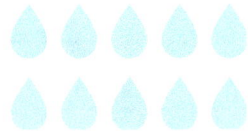

Biggest Learning:

Today's Magic Moment:

Daily
Plan

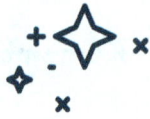

Day at a glance

6 am	
7 am	
8 am	
9 am	
10 am	
11 am	
12 pm	
1 pm	
2 pm	
3 pm	
4 pm	
5 pm	
6 pm	
7 pm	

Top Priorities!

Glass of Water Score

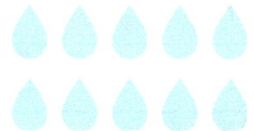

Biggest Learning:

Today's Magic Moment:

Monthly

Focus

Goals	Due By

Tasks

- [ ]
- [ ]
- [ ]
- [ ]
- [ ]
- [ ]

Results

Weekly Snapshot

Week Commencing:

New Habit
Name It.

Must Do This Week!

Track It.

- ☐ Mon
- ☐ Tues
- ☐ Wed
- ☐ Thurs
- ☐ Fri
- ☐ Sat
- ☐ Sun

Quote For The Week:

Nothing is more intolerable than to have to admit to yourself your own errors.

BEETHOVEN

Review It.
How did it go?
What worked?
What didn't?

Daily
Plan

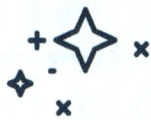

Day at a glance

Remember This!

6 am	
7 am	
8 am	
9 am	
10 am	
11 am	
12 pm	
1 pm	
2 pm	
3 pm	
4 pm	
5 pm	
6 pm	
7 pm	

Top Priorities!

Glass of Water Score

Biggest Learning:

Today's Magic Moment:

Daily
Plan

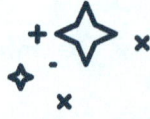

Day at a glance

6 am	
7 am	
8 am	
9 am	
10 am	
11 am	
12 pm	
1 pm	
2 pm	
3 pm	
4 pm	
5 pm	
6 pm	
7 pm	

Top Priorities!

Glass of Water Score

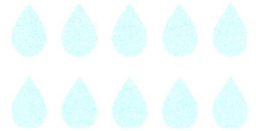

Biggest Learning:

Today's Magic Moment:

Daily Plan

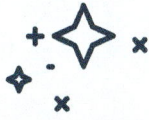

Day at a glance

6 am	
7 am	
8 am	
9 am	
10 am	
11 am	
12 pm	
1 pm	
2 pm	
3 pm	
4 pm	
5 pm	
6 pm	
7 pm	

Remember This!

Top Priorities!

Glass of Water Score

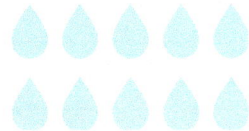

Biggest Learning:

Today's Magic Moment:

Daily Plan

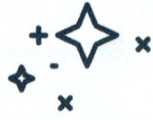

Day at a glance

6 am	
7 am	
8 am	
9 am	
10 am	
11 am	
12 pm	
1 pm	
2 pm	
3 pm	
4 pm	
5 pm	
6 pm	
7 pm	

Remember This!

Top Priorities!

Glass of Water Score

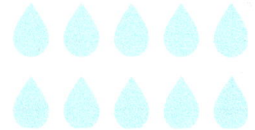

Biggest Learning:

Today's Magic Moment:

Daily
Plan

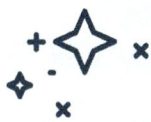

Day at a glance

Remember This!

6 am	
7 am	
8 am	
9 am	
10 am	
11 am	
12 pm	
1 pm	
2 pm	
3 pm	
4 pm	
5 pm	
6 pm	
7 pm	

Top Priorities!

Glass of Water Score

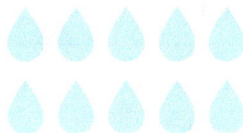

Biggest Learning:

Today's Magic Moment:

Daily

Plan

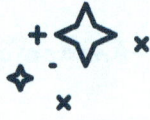

Day at a glance

6 am	
7 am	
8 am	
9 am	
10 am	
11 am	
12 pm	
1 pm	
2 pm	
3 pm	
4 pm	
5 pm	
6 pm	
7 pm	

Top Priorities!

Glass of Water Score

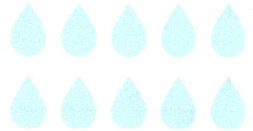

Biggest Learning:

Today's Magic Moment:

Daily Plan

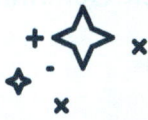

Day at a glance

6 am	
7 am	
8 am	
9 am	
10 am	
11 am	
12 pm	
1 pm	
2 pm	
3 pm	
4 pm	
5 pm	
6 pm	
7 pm	

Remember This!

Top Priorities!

Glass of Water Score

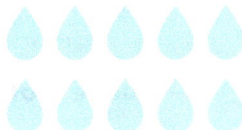

Biggest Learning:

Today's Magic Moment:

Weekly Snapshot

Week Commencing:

New Habit

Name It.

Must Do This Week!

Track It.

☐   Mon

☐   Tues

☐   Wed

☐   Thurs

☐   Fri

☐   Sat

☐   Sun

Quote For The Week:

You are braver than you
Believe.

Stronger than you seem.

Smarter than you think.

And Loved more than you'll
ever know.

WINNIE THE POO

Review It.
How did it go?
What worked?
What didn't?

Daily
Plan

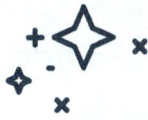

Day at a glance

6 am	
7 am	
8 am	
9 am	
10 am	
11 am	
12 pm	
1 pm	
2 pm	
3 pm	
4 pm	
5 pm	
6 pm	
7 pm	

Top Priorities!

Glass of Water Score

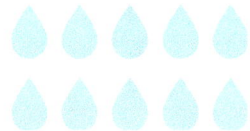

Biggest Learning:

Today's Magic Moment:

Daily Plan

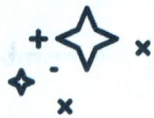

Day at a glance

6 am	
7 am	
8 am	
9 am	
10 am	
11 am	
12 pm	
1 pm	
2 pm	
3 pm	
4 pm	
5 pm	
6 pm	
7 pm	

Remember This!

Top Priorities!

Glass of Water Score

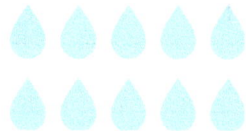

Biggest Learning:

Today's Magic Moment:

Daily
Plan

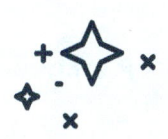

Day at a glance

6 am	
7 am	
8 am	
9 am	
10 am	
11 am	
12 pm	
1 pm	
2 pm	
3 pm	
4 pm	
5 pm	
6 pm	
7 pm	

Top Priorities!

Glass of Water Score

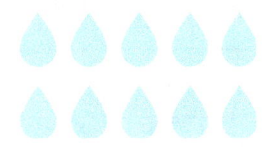

💧💧💧💧💧
💧💧💧💧💧

Biggest Learning:

Today's Magic Moment:

Daily Plan

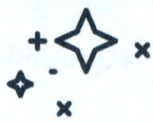

Day at a glance

6 am	
7 am	
8 am	
9 am	
10 am	
11 am	
12 pm	
1 pm	
2 pm	
3 pm	
4 pm	
5 pm	
6 pm	
7 pm	

Remember This!

Top Priorities!

Glass of Water Score

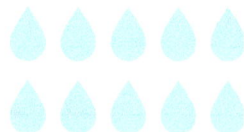

Biggest Learning:

Today's Magic Moment:

Daily Plan

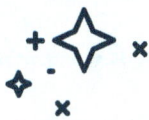

Day at a glance

6 am	
7 am	
8 am	
9 am	
10 am	
11 am	
12 pm	
1 pm	
2 pm	
3 pm	
4 pm	
5 pm	
6 pm	
7 pm	

Remember This!

Top Priorities!

Glass of Water Score

Biggest Learning:

Today's Magic Moment:

Daily

Plan

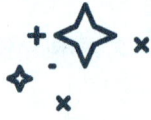

Day at a glance

6 am	
7 am	
8 am	
9 am	
10 am	
11 am	
12 pm	
1 pm	
2 pm	
3 pm	
4 pm	
5 pm	
6 pm	
7 pm	

Top Priorities!

Glass of Water Score

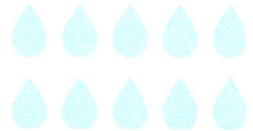

Biggest Learning:

Today's Magic Moment:

Daily

Plan

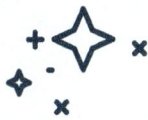

Day at a glance

6 am	
7 am	
8 am	
9 am	
10 am	
11 am	
12 pm	
1 pm	
2 pm	
3 pm	
4 pm	
5 pm	
6 pm	
7 pm	

Remember This!

Top Priorities!

Glass of Water Score

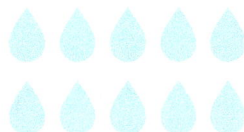

Biggest Learning:

Today's Magic Moment:

Weekly Snapshot

New Habit

Name It.

Must Do This Week!

Track It.

- ☐ Mon
- ☐ Tues
- ☐ Wed
- ☐ Thurs
- ☐ Fri
- ☐ Sat
- ☐ Sun

Quote For The Week:

What we wish,
we readily believe,
and what we ourselves think,
we imagine others think also.

JULIUS CAESAR

Review It.
How did it go?
What worked?
What didn't?

Daily Plan

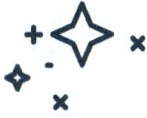

Day at a glance

6 am	
7 am	
8 am	
9 am	
10 am	
11 am	
12 pm	
1 pm	
2 pm	
3 pm	
4 pm	
5 pm	
6 pm	
7 pm	

Top Priorities!

Glass of Water Score

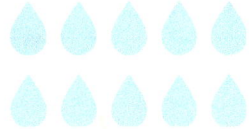

Biggest Learning:

Today's Magic Moment:

Daily Plan

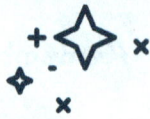

Day at a glance

6 am	
7 am	
8 am	
9 am	
10 am	
11 am	
12 pm	
1 pm	
2 pm	
3 pm	
4 pm	
5 pm	
6 pm	
7 pm	

Remember This!

Top Priorities!

Glass of Water Score

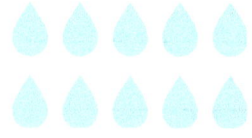

Biggest Learning:

Today's Magic Moment:

Daily Plan

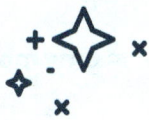

Day at a glance

6 am	
7 am	
8 am	
9 am	
10 am	
11 am	
12 pm	
1 pm	
2 pm	
3 pm	
4 pm	
5 pm	
6 pm	
7 pm	

Remember This!

Top Priorities!

Glass of Water Score

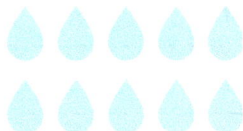

Biggest Learning:

Today's Magic Moment:

Daily Plan

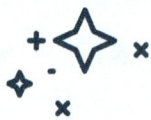

Day at a glance

Remember This!

6 am	
7 am	
8 am	
9 am	
10 am	
11 am	
12 pm	
1 pm	
2 pm	
3 pm	
4 pm	
5 pm	
6 pm	
7 pm	

Top Priorities!

Glass of Water Score

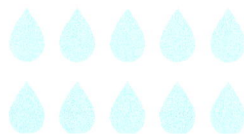

Biggest Learning:

Today's Magic Moment:

Daily Plan

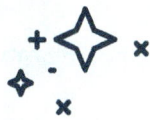

Day at a glance

6 am	
7 am	
8 am	
9 am	
10 am	
11 am	
12 pm	
1 pm	
2 pm	
3 pm	
4 pm	
5 pm	
6 pm	
7 pm	

Remember This!

Top Priorities!

Glass of Water Score

Biggest Learning:

Today's Magic Moment:

Daily
Plan
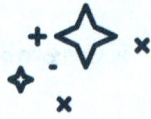

Day at a glance

Time	
6 am	
7 am	
8 am	
9 am	
10 am	
11 am	
12 pm	
1 pm	
2 pm	
3 pm	
4 pm	
5 pm	
6 pm	
7 pm	

Remember This!

Top Priorities!

Glass of Water Score

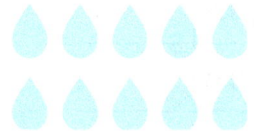

Biggest Learning:

Today's Magic Moment:

Daily

Plan

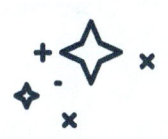

Day at a glance

6 am	
7 am	
8 am	
9 am	
10 am	
11 am	
12 pm	
1 pm	
2 pm	
3 pm	
4 pm	
5 pm	
6 pm	
7 pm	

Remember This!

Top Priorities!

Glass of Water Score

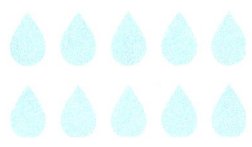

Biggest Learning:

Today's Magic Moment:

Weekly Snapshot

Week Commencing:

New Habit
Name It.

Must Do This Week!

Track It.

- ☐ Mon
- ☐ Tues
- ☐ Wed
- ☐ Thurs
- ☐ Fri
- ☐ Sat
- ☐ Sun

Quote For The Week:

Review It.
How did it go?
What worked?
What didn't?

Daily
Plan

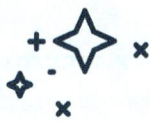

Day at a glance

6 am	
7 am	
8 am	
9 am	
10 am	
11 am	
12 pm	
1 pm	
2 pm	
3 pm	
4 pm	
5 pm	
6 pm	
7 pm	

Remember This!

Top Priorities!

Glass of Water Score

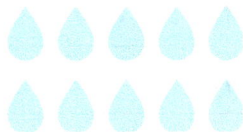

Biggest Learning:

Today's Magic Moment:

Daily
Plan

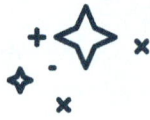

Day at a glance

6 am	
7 am	
8 am	
9 am	
10 am	
11 am	
12 pm	
1 pm	
2 pm	
3 pm	
4 pm	
5 pm	
6 pm	
7 pm	

Top Priorities!

Glass of Water Score

Biggest Learning:

Today's Magic Moment:

Daily Plan

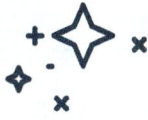

Day at a glance

6 am	
7 am	
8 am	
9 am	
10 am	
11 am	
12 pm	
1 pm	
2 pm	
3 pm	
4 pm	
5 pm	
6 pm	
7 pm	

Remember This!

Top Priorities!

Glass of Water Score

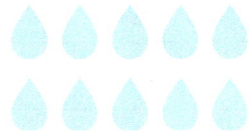

Biggest Learning:

Today's Magic Moment:

Daily
Plan

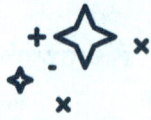

Day at a glance

6 am	
7 am	
8 am	
9 am	
10 am	
11 am	
12 pm	
1 pm	
2 pm	
3 pm	
4 pm	
5 pm	
6 pm	
7 pm	

Top Priorities!

Glass of Water Score

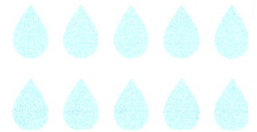

Biggest Learning:

Today's Magic Moment:

Daily

Plan

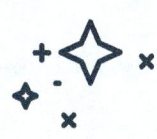

Day at a glance

6 am	
7 am	
8 am	
9 am	
10 am	
11 am	
12 pm	
1 pm	
2 pm	
3 pm	
4 pm	
5 pm	
6 pm	
7 pm	

Remember This!

Top Priorities!

Glass of Water Score

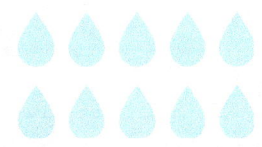

Biggest Learning:

Today's Magic Moment:

Daily

Plan

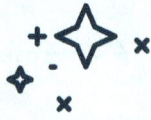

Day at a glance

6 am	
7 am	
8 am	
9 am	
10 am	
11 am	
12 pm	
1 pm	
2 pm	
3 pm	
4 pm	
5 pm	
6 pm	
7 pm	

Biggest Learning:

Remember This!

Top Priorities!

Glass of Water Score

Today's Magic Moment:

Daily

Plan

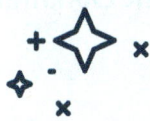

Day at a glance

6 am	
7 am	
8 am	
9 am	
10 am	
11 am	
12 pm	
1 pm	
2 pm	
3 pm	
4 pm	
5 pm	
6 pm	
7 pm	

Remember This!

Top Priorities!

Glass of Water Score

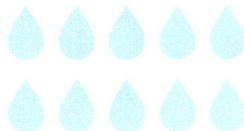

Biggest Learning:

Today's Magic Moment:

Weekly Snapshot

Week Commencing:

New Habit

Name It.

Must Do This Week!

Track It.

- ☐ Mon
- ☐ Tues
- ☐ Wed
- ☐ Thurs
- ☐ Fri
- ☐ Sat
- ☐ Sun

Quote For The Week:

Whatever you're meant to do,

do it now.

The conditions are always
impossible.

DORIS LESSING

Review It.

How did it go?
What worked?
What didn't?

Daily
Plan

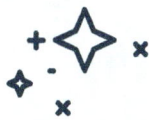

Day at a glance

6 am	
7 am	
8 am	
9 am	
10 am	
11 am	
12 pm	
1 pm	
2 pm	
3 pm	
4 pm	
5 pm	
6 pm	
7 pm	

Top Priorities!

Glass of Water Score

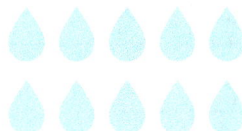

💧💧💧💧💧
💧💧💧💧💧

Biggest Learning:

Today's Magic Moment:

Daily Plan

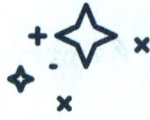

Day at a glance

6 am	
7 am	
8 am	
9 am	
10 am	
11 am	
12 pm	
1 pm	
2 pm	
3 pm	
4 pm	
5 pm	
6 pm	
7 pm	

Remember This!

Top Priorities!

Glass of Water Score

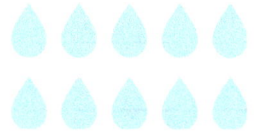

Biggest Learning:

Today's Magic Moment:

Daily Plan

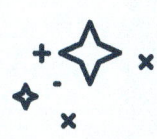

Day at a glance

Time	
6 am	
7 am	
8 am	
9 am	
10 am	
11 am	
12 pm	
1 pm	
2 pm	
3 pm	
4 pm	
5 pm	
6 pm	
7 pm	

Remember This!

Top Priorities!

Glass of Water Score

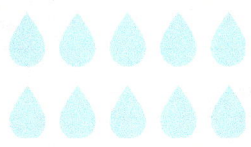

Biggest Learning:

Today's Magic Moment:

Daily Plan

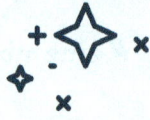

Day at a glance

6 am	
7 am	
8 am	
9 am	
10 am	
11 am	
12 pm	
1 pm	
2 pm	
3 pm	
4 pm	
5 pm	
6 pm	
7 pm	

Remember This!

Top Priorities!

Glass of Water Score

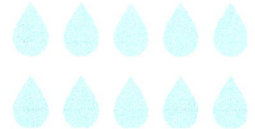

Biggest Learning:

Today's Magic Moment:

Daily Plan

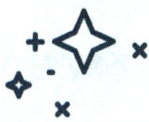

Day at a glance

6 am	
7 am	
8 am	
9 am	
10 am	
11 am	
12 pm	
1 pm	
2 pm	
3 pm	
4 pm	
5 pm	
6 pm	
7 pm	

Remember This!

Top Priorities!

Glass of Water Score

Biggest Learning:

Today's Magic Moment:

Daily Plan

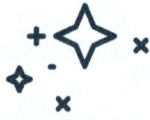

Day at a glance

6 am	
7 am	
8 am	
9 am	
10 am	
11 am	
12 pm	
1 pm	
2 pm	
3 pm	
4 pm	
5 pm	
6 pm	
7 pm	

Remember This!

Top Priorities!

Glass of Water Score

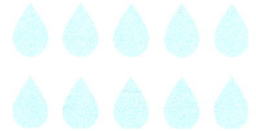

Biggest Learning:

Today's Magic Moment:

Daily Plan

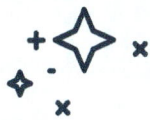

Day at a glance

6 am	
7 am	
8 am	
9 am	
10 am	
11 am	
12 pm	
1 pm	
2 pm	
3 pm	
4 pm	
5 pm	
6 pm	
7 pm	

Remember This!

Top Priorities!

Glass of Water Score

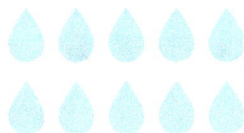

Biggest Learning:

Today's Magic Moment:

Monthly

Focus

Goals   Due By

_____   _____

_____   _____

_____   _____

_____   _____

_____   _____

_____   _____

_____   _____

| |

Tasks

Results

☐ _____

☐ _____

☐ _____

☐ _____

☐ _____

☐ _____

Weekly
Snapshot

Week Commencing:

Must Do This Week!

New Habit

Name It.

Track It.

- ☐ Mon
- ☐ Tues
- ☐ Wed
- ☐ Thurs
- ☐ Fri
- ☐ Sat
- ☐ Sun

Quote For The Week:

First say to yourself what
you would be;
and then do
what you have to do.

EPICTETUS

Review It.
How did it go?
What worked?
What didn't?

Daily Plan

Day at a glance

6 am	
7 am	
8 am	
9 am	
10 am	
11 am	
12 pm	
1 pm	
2 pm	
3 pm	
4 pm	
5 pm	
6 pm	
7 pm	

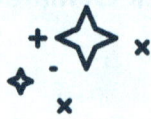

Remember This!

Top Priorities!

Glass of Water Score

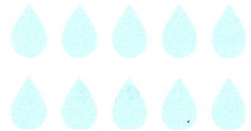

Biggest Learning:

Today's Magic Moment:

Daily
Plan

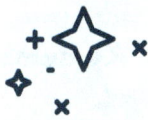

Day at a glance

6 am	
7 am	
8 am	
9 am	
10 am	
11 am	
12 pm	
1 pm	
2 pm	
3 pm	
4 pm	
5 pm	
6 pm	
7 pm	

Top Priorities!

Glass of Water Score

💧💧💧💧💧
💧💧💧💧💧

Biggest Learning:

Today's Magic Moment:

Daily
Plan

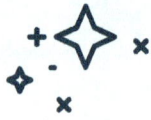

Day at a glance

6 am	
7 am	
8 am	
9 am	
10 am	
11 am	
12 pm	
1 pm	
2 pm	
3 pm	
4 pm	
5 pm	
6 pm	
7 pm	

Top Priorities!

Glass of Water Score

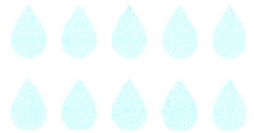

Biggest Learning:

Today's Magic Moment:

Daily Plan

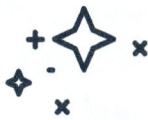

Day at a glance

6 am	
7 am	
8 am	
9 am	
10 am	
11 am	
12 pm	
1 pm	
2 pm	
3 pm	
4 pm	
5 pm	
6 pm	
7 pm	

Top Priorities!

Glass of Water Score

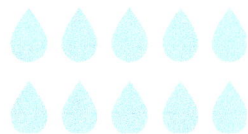

Biggest Learning:

Today's Magic Moment:

Daily Plan

Day at a glance

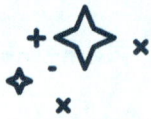

Remember This!

6 am	
7 am	
8 am	
9 am	
10 am	
11 am	
12 pm	
1 pm	
2 pm	
3 pm	
4 pm	
5 pm	
6 pm	
7 pm	

Top Priorities!

Glass of Water Score

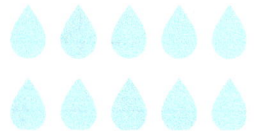

Biggest Learning:

Today's Magic Moment:

Daily

Plan

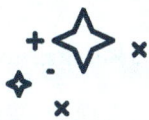

Day at a glance

6 am	
7 am	
8 am	
9 am	
10 am	
11 am	
12 pm	
1 pm	
2 pm	
3 pm	
4 pm	
5 pm	
6 pm	
7 pm	

Top Priorities!

Glass of Water Score

Biggest Learning:

Today's Magic Moment:

Daily Plan

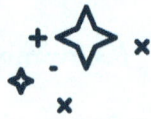

Day at a glance

Time	
6 am	
7 am	
8 am	
9 am	
10 am	
11 am	
12 pm	
1 pm	
2 pm	
3 pm	
4 pm	
5 pm	
6 pm	
7 pm	

Remember This!

Top Priorities!

Glass of Water Score

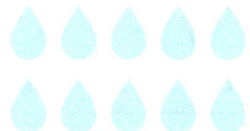

Biggest Learning:

Today's Magic Moment:

Weekly Snapshot

Week Commencing:

Must Do This Week!

New Habit

Name It.

Track It.

☐ Mon

☐ Tues

☐ Wed

☐ Thurs

☐ Fri

☐ Sat

☐ Sun

Quote For The Week:

Review It.
How did it go?
What worked?
What didn't?

Daily Plan

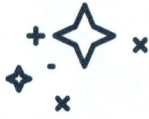

Day at a glance

6 am	
7 am	
8 am	
9 am	
10 am	
11 am	
12 pm	
1 pm	
2 pm	
3 pm	
4 pm	
5 pm	
6 pm	
7 pm	

Remember This!

Top Priorities!

Glass of Water Score

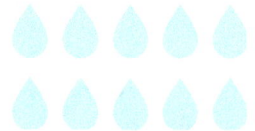

Biggest Learning:

Today's Magic Moment:

Daily Plan

Day at a glance

6 am	
7 am	
8 am	
9 am	
10 am	
11 am	
12 pm	
1 pm	
2 pm	
3 pm	
4 pm	
5 pm	
6 pm	
7 pm	

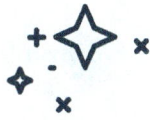

Remember This!

Top Priorities!

Glass of Water Score

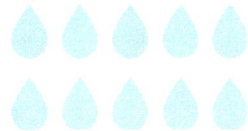

Biggest Learning:

Today's Magic Moment:

Daily Plan

Day at a glance

6 am	
7 am	
8 am	
9 am	
10 am	
11 am	
12 pm	
1 pm	
2 pm	
3 pm	
4 pm	
5 pm	
6 pm	
7 pm	

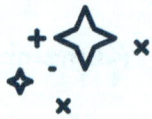

Remember This!

Top Priorities!

Glass of Water Score

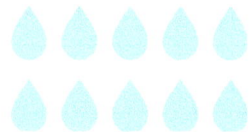

Biggest Learning:

Today's Magic Moment:

Daily Plan

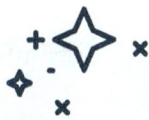

Day at a glance

Time	
6 am	
7 am	
8 am	
9 am	
10 am	
11 am	
12 pm	
1 pm	
2 pm	
3 pm	
4 pm	
5 pm	
6 pm	
7 pm	

Remember This!

Top Priorities!

Glass of Water Score

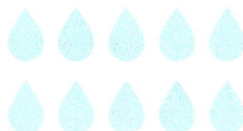

💧💧💧💧💧
💧💧💧💧💧

Biggest Learning:

Today's Magic Moment:

Daily Plan

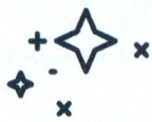

Day at a glance

6 am	
7 am	
8 am	
9 am	
10 am	
11 am	
12 pm	
1 pm	
2 pm	
3 pm	
4 pm	
5 pm	
6 pm	
7 pm	

Remember This!

Top Priorities!

Glass of Water Score

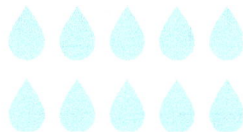

Biggest Learning:

Today's Magic Moment:

Daily Plan

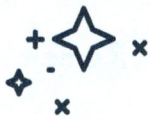

Day at a glance

Time	
6 am	
7 am	
8 am	
9 am	
10 am	
11 am	
12 pm	
1 pm	
2 pm	
3 pm	
4 pm	
5 pm	
6 pm	
7 pm	

Remember This!

Top Priorities!

Glass of Water Score

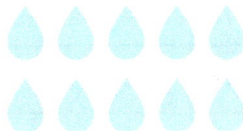

Biggest Learning:

Today's Magic Moment:

Daily
Plan

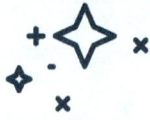

Day at a glance

6 am	
7 am	
8 am	
9 am	
10 am	
11 am	
12 pm	
1 pm	
2 pm	
3 pm	
4 pm	
5 pm	
6 pm	
7 pm	

Top Priorities!

Glass of Water Score

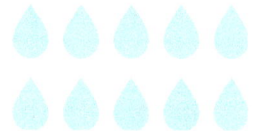

Biggest Learning:

Today's Magic Moment:

Weekly
Snapshot

Week Commencing:

New Habit

Name It.

Must Do This Week!

Track It.

☐   Mon

☐   Tues

☐   Wed

☐   Thurs

☐   Fri

☐   Sat

Quote For The Week:

☐   Sun

Review It.
How did it go?
What worked?
What didn't?

Pleasure in the job

puts perfection in the work.

ARISTOTLE

Daily Plan

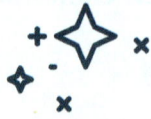

Day at a glance

6 am	
7 am	
8 am	
9 am	
10 am	
11 am	
12 pm	
1 pm	
2 pm	
3 pm	
4 pm	
5 pm	
6 pm	
7 pm	

Remember This!

Top Priorities!

Glass of Water Score

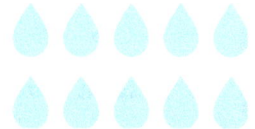

Biggest Learning:

Today's Magic Moment:

Daily

Plan

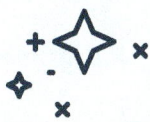

Day at a glance

6 am	
7 am	
8 am	
9 am	
10 am	
11 am	
12 pm	
1 pm	
2 pm	
3 pm	
4 pm	
5 pm	
6 pm	
7 pm	

Remember This!

Top Priorities!

Glass of Water Score

Biggest Learning:

Today's Magic Moment:

Daily
Plan

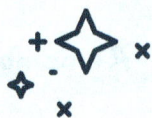

Day at a glance

6 am	
7 am	
8 am	
9 am	
10 am	
11 am	
12 pm	
1 pm	
2 pm	
3 pm	
4 pm	
5 pm	
6 pm	
7 pm	

Remember This!

Top Priorities!

Glass of Water Score

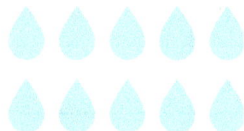

Biggest Learning:

Today's Magic Moment:

Daily

Plan

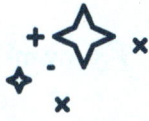

Day at a glance

6 am	
7 am	
8 am	
9 am	
10 am	
11 am	
12 pm	
1 pm	
2 pm	
3 pm	
4 pm	
5 pm	
6 pm	
7 pm	

Remember This!

Top Priorities!

Glass of Water Score

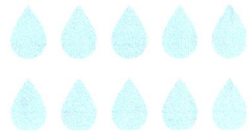

Biggest Learning:

Today's Magic Moment:

Daily
Plan

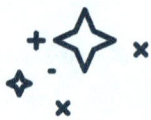

Day at a glance

6 am	
7 am	
8 am	
9 am	
10 am	
11 am	
12 pm	
1 pm	
2 pm	
3 pm	
4 pm	
5 pm	
6 pm	
7 pm	

Top Priorities!

Glass of Water Score

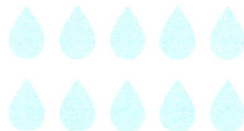

Biggest Learning:

Today's Magic Moment:

Daily
Plan

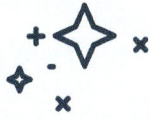

Day at a glance

6 am	
7 am	
8 am	
9 am	
10 am	
11 am	
12 pm	
1 pm	
2 pm	
3 pm	
4 pm	
5 pm	
6 pm	
7 pm	

Remember This!

Top Priorities!

Glass of Water Score

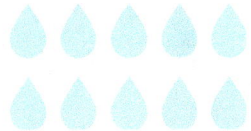

Biggest Learning:

Today's Magic Moment:

Daily Plan

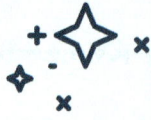

Day at a glance

6 am	
7 am	
8 am	
9 am	
10 am	
11 am	
12 pm	
1 pm	
2 pm	
3 pm	
4 pm	
5 pm	
6 pm	
7 pm	

Remember This!

Top Priorities!

Glass of Water Score

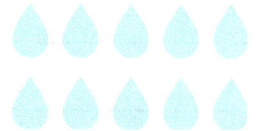

Biggest Learning:

Today's Magic Moment:

Weekly Snapshot

New Habit

Name It.

Must Do This Week!

Track It.

- ☐ Mon
- ☐ Tues
- ☐ Wed
- ☐ Thurs
- ☐ Fri
- ☐ Sat
- ☐ Sun

Quote For The Week:

Courage isn't having the strength to go on - it is going on when you don't have strength.

NAPOLEON BONAPARTE

Review It.
How did it go?
What worked?
What didn't?

Daily
Plan

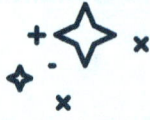

Day at a glance

6 am	
7 am	
8 am	
9 am	
10 am	
11 am	
12 pm	
1 pm	
2 pm	
3 pm	
4 pm	
5 pm	
6 pm	
7 pm	

Top Priorities!

Glass of Water Score

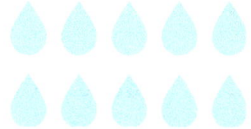

Biggest Learning:

Today's Magic Moment:

Daily
Plan

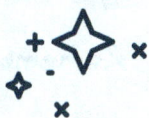

Day at a glance

6 am	
7 am	
8 am	
9 am	
10 am	
11 am	
12 pm	
1 pm	
2 pm	
3 pm	
4 pm	
5 pm	
6 pm	
7 pm	

Remember This!

Top Priorities!

Glass of Water Score

Biggest Learning:

Today's Magic Moment:

Daily Plan

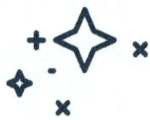

Day at a glance

6 am	
7 am	
8 am	
9 am	
10 am	
11 am	
12 pm	
1 pm	
2 pm	
3 pm	
4 pm	
5 pm	
6 pm	
7 pm	

Remember This!

Top Priorities!

Glass of Water Score

Biggest Learning:

Today's Magic Moment:

Daily
Plan

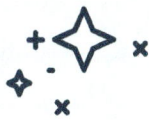

Day at a glance

6 am	
7 am	
8 am	
9 am	
10 am	
11 am	
12 pm	
1 pm	
2 pm	
3 pm	
4 pm	
5 pm	
6 pm	
7 pm	

Top Priorities!

Glass of Water Score

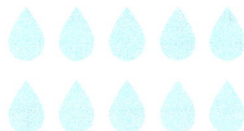

💧💧💧💧💧
💧💧💧💧💧

Biggest Learning:

Today's Magic Moment:

Daily Plan

Day at a glance

6 am	
7 am	
8 am	
9 am	
10 am	
11 am	
12 pm	
1 pm	
2 pm	
3 pm	
4 pm	
5 pm	
6 pm	
7 pm	

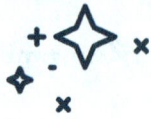

Remember This!

Top Priorities!

Glass of Water Score

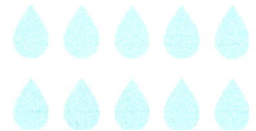

Biggest Learning:

Today's Magic Moment:

Daily Plan

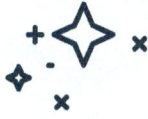

Day at a glance

6 am	
7 am	
8 am	
9 am	
10 am	
11 am	
12 pm	
1 pm	
2 pm	
3 pm	
4 pm	
5 pm	
6 pm	
7 pm	

Remember This!

Top Priorities!

Glass of Water Score

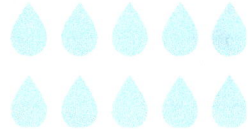

Biggest Learning:

Today's Magic Moment:

Daily
Plan

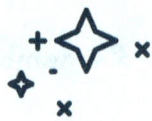

Day at a glance

6 am	
7 am	
8 am	
9 am	
10 am	
11 am	
12 pm	
1 pm	
2 pm	
3 pm	
4 pm	
5 pm	
6 pm	
7 pm	

Top Priorities!

Glass of Water Score

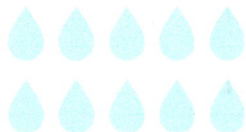

Biggest Learning:

Today's Magic Moment:

Weekly Snapshot

Must Do This Week!

Quote For The Week:

New Habit

Name It.

Track It.

☐ Mon

☐ Tues

☐ Wed

☐ Thurs

☐ Fri

☐ Sat

☐ Sun

Review It.
How did it go?
What worked?
What didn't?

Daily Plan

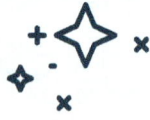

Day at a glance

6 am	
7 am	
8 am	
9 am	
10 am	
11 am	
12 pm	
1 pm	
2 pm	
3 pm	
4 pm	
5 pm	
6 pm	
7 pm	

Remember This!

Top Priorities!

Glass of Water Score

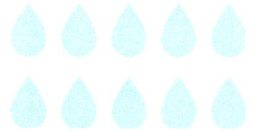

Biggest Learning:

Today's Magic Moment:

Daily Plan

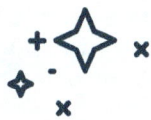

Day at a glance

6 am	
7 am	
8 am	
9 am	
10 am	
11 am	
12 pm	
1 pm	
2 pm	
3 pm	
4 pm	
5 pm	
6 pm	
7 pm	

Remember This!

Top Priorities!

Glass of Water Score

Biggest Learning:

Today's Magic Moment:

Daily Plan

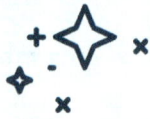

Day at a glance

6 am	
7 am	
8 am	
9 am	
10 am	
11 am	
12 pm	
1 pm	
2 pm	
3 pm	
4 pm	
5 pm	
6 pm	
7 pm	

Remember This!

Top Priorities!

Glass of Water Score

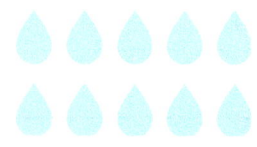

Biggest Learning:

Today's Magic Moment:

Daily
Plan

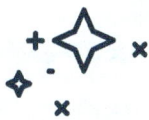

Day at a glance

6 am	
7 am	
8 am	
9 am	
10 am	
11 am	
12 pm	
1 pm	
2 pm	
3 pm	
4 pm	
5 pm	
6 pm	
7 pm	

Remember This!

Top Priorities!

Glass of Water Score

Biggest Learning:

Today's Magic Moment:

Daily Plan

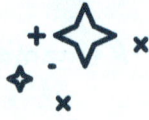

Day at a glance

6 am	
7 am	
8 am	
9 am	
10 am	
11 am	
12 pm	
1 pm	
2 pm	
3 pm	
4 pm	
5 pm	
6 pm	
7 pm	

Top Priorities!

Glass of Water Score

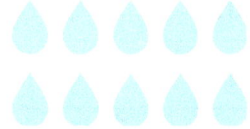

Biggest Learning:

Today's Magic Moment:

Daily
Plan

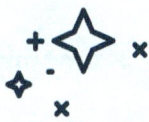

Day at a glance

6 am	
7 am	
8 am	
9 am	
10 am	
11 am	
12 pm	
1 pm	
2 pm	
3 pm	
4 pm	
5 pm	
6 pm	
7 pm	

Remember This!

Top Priorities!

Glass of Water Score

Biggest Learning:

Today's Magic Moment:

Daily Plan

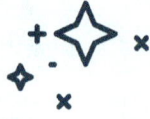

Day at a glance

6 am	
7 am	
8 am	
9 am	
10 am	
11 am	
12 pm	
1 pm	
2 pm	
3 pm	
4 pm	
5 pm	
6 pm	
7 pm	

Top Priorities!

Glass of Water Score

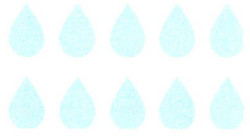

Biggest Learning:

Today's Magic Moment:

Monthly

Focus

Goals	Due By

Results

Tasks

- [ ]
- [ ]
- [ ]
- [ ]
- [ ]
- [ ]

Weekly Snapshot

New Habit

Name It.

Must Do This Week!

Track It.

- ☐ Mon
- ☐ Tues
- ☐ Wed
- ☐ Thurs
- ☐ Fri
- ☐ Sat
- ☐ Sun

Quote For The Week:

Good character is not formed in a week or a month. It is created little by little, day by day. Protracted and patient effort is needed to develop good character.

HERACLITUS

Review It.
How did it go?
What worked?
What didn't?

Daily Plan

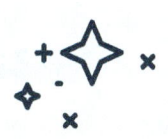

Day at a glance

6 am	
7 am	
8 am	
9 am	
10 am	
11 am	
12 pm	
1 pm	
2 pm	
3 pm	
4 pm	
5 pm	
6 pm	
7 pm	

Remember This!

Top Priorities!

Glass of Water Score

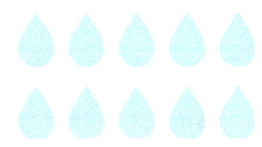

Biggest Learning:

Today's Magic Moment:

Daily Plan

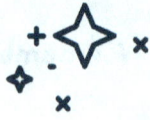

Day at a glance

6 am	
7 am	
8 am	
9 am	
10 am	
11 am	
12 pm	
1 pm	
2 pm	
3 pm	
4 pm	
5 pm	
6 pm	
7 pm	

Remember This!

Top Priorities!

Glass of Water Score

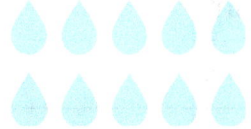

Biggest Learning:

Today's Magic Moment:

Daily Plan

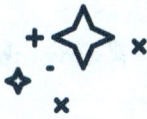

Day at a glance

6 am	
7 am	
8 am	
9 am	
10 am	
11 am	
12 pm	
1 pm	
2 pm	
3 pm	
4 pm	
5 pm	
6 pm	
7 pm	

Remember This!

Top Priorities!

Glass of Water Score

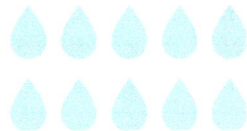

Biggest Learning:

Today's Magic Moment:

Daily
Plan

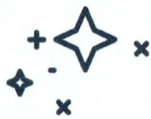

Day at a glance

6 am	
7 am	
8 am	
9 am	
10 am	
11 am	
12 pm	
1 pm	
2 pm	
3 pm	
4 pm	
5 pm	
6 pm	
7 pm	

Top Priorities!

Glass of Water Score

💧💧💧💧💧
💧💧💧💧💧

Biggest Learning:

Today's Magic Moment:

Daily Plan

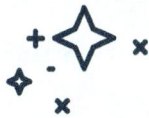

Day at a glance

6 am	
7 am	
8 am	
9 am	
10 am	
11 am	
12 pm	
1 pm	
2 pm	
3 pm	
4 pm	
5 pm	
6 pm	
7 pm	

Remember This!

Top Priorities!

Glass of Water Score

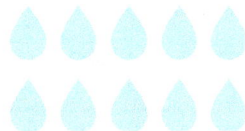

Biggest Learning:

Today's Magic Moment:

Daily

Plan

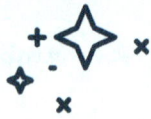

Day at a glance

6 am	
7 am	
8 am	
9 am	
10 am	
11 am	
12 pm	
1 pm	
2 pm	
3 pm	
4 pm	
5 pm	
6 pm	
7 pm	

Top Priorities!

Glass of Water Score

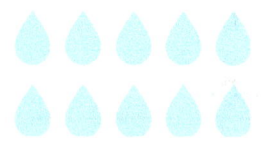

💧💧💧💧💧

💧💧💧💧💧

Biggest Learning:

Today's Magic Moment:

Daily
Plan

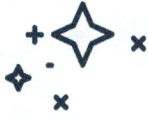

Day at a glance

6 am	
7 am	
8 am	
9 am	
10 am	
11 am	
12 pm	
1 pm	
2 pm	
3 pm	
4 pm	
5 pm	
6 pm	
7 pm	

Remember This!

Top Priorities!

Glass of Water Score

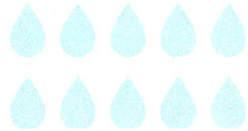

Biggest Learning:

Today's Magic Moment:

Weekly Snapshot

Week Commencing:

New Habit

Name It.

Must Do This Week!

Track It.

☐ Mon

☐ Tues

☐ Wed

☐ Thurs

☐ Fri

☐ Sat

☐ Sun

Quote For The Week:

Review It.
How did it go?
What worked?
What didn't?

Daily Plan

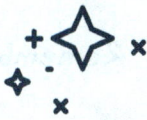

Day at a glance

6 am	
7 am	
8 am	
9 am	
10 am	
11 am	
12 pm	
1 pm	
2 pm	
3 pm	
4 pm	
5 pm	
6 pm	
7 pm	

Remember This!

Top Priorities!

Glass of Water Score

Biggest Learning:

Today's Magic Moment:

Daily Plan

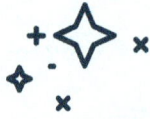

Day at a glance

6 am	
7 am	
8 am	
9 am	
10 am	
11 am	
12 pm	
1 pm	
2 pm	
3 pm	
4 pm	
5 pm	
6 pm	
7 pm	

Remember This!

Top Priorities!

Glass of Water Score

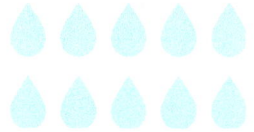

Biggest Learning:

Today's Magic Moment:

Daily Plan

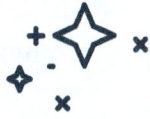

Day at a glance

Time	
6 am	
7 am	
8 am	
9 am	
10 am	
11 am	
12 pm	
1 pm	
2 pm	
3 pm	
4 pm	
5 pm	
6 pm	
7 pm	

Remember This!

Top Priorities!

Glass of Water Score

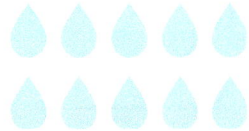

Biggest Learning:

Today's Magic Moment:

Daily Plan

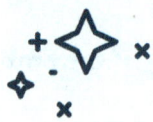

Day at a glance

Time	
6 am	
7 am	
8 am	
9 am	
10 am	
11 am	
12 pm	
1 pm	
2 pm	
3 pm	
4 pm	
5 pm	
6 pm	
7 pm	

Remember This!

Top Priorities!

Glass of Water Score

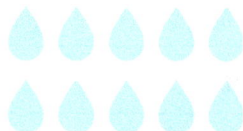

Biggest Learning:

Today's Magic Moment:

Daily Plan

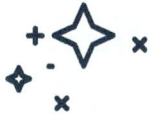

Day at a glance

Time	
6 am	
7 am	
8 am	
9 am	
10 am	
11 am	
12 pm	
1 pm	
2 pm	
3 pm	
4 pm	
5 pm	
6 pm	
7 pm	

Remember This!

Top Priorities!

Glass of Water Score

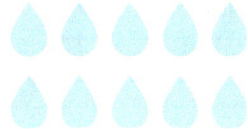

Biggest Learning:

Today's Magic Moment:

Daily Plan

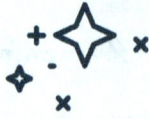

Day at a glance

Time	
6 am	
7 am	
8 am	
9 am	
10 am	
11 am	
12 pm	
1 pm	
2 pm	
3 pm	
4 pm	
5 pm	
6 pm	
7 pm	

Remember This!

Top Priorities!

Glass of Water Score

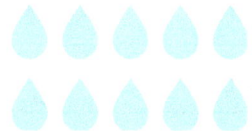

Biggest Learning:

Today's Magic Moment:

Daily Plan

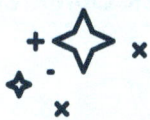

Day at a glance

Time	
6 am	
7 am	
8 am	
9 am	
10 am	
11 am	
12 pm	
1 pm	
2 pm	
3 pm	
4 pm	
5 pm	
6 pm	
7 pm	

Remember This!

Top Priorities!

Glass of Water Score

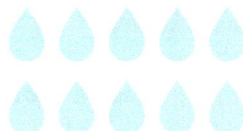

Biggest Learning:

Today's Magic Moment:

Weekly Snapshot

Week Commencing:

New Habit
Name It.

Must Do This Week!

Track It.

- ☐ Mon
- ☐ Tues
- ☐ Wed
- ☐ Thurs
- ☐ Fri
- ☐ Sat
- ☐ Sun

Quote For The Week:

Wherever you go,

no matter what the weather,

always bring your own sunshine.

ANTHONY J. D'ANGELO

Review It.
How did it go?
What worked?
What didn't?

Daily Plan

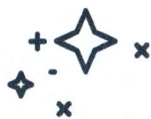

Day at a glance

6 am	
7 am	
8 am	
9 am	
10 am	
11 am	
12 pm	
1 pm	
2 pm	
3 pm	
4 pm	
5 pm	
6 pm	
7 pm	

Remember This!

Top Priorities!

Glass of Water Score

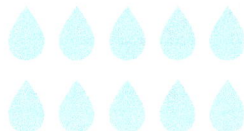

Biggest Learning:

Today's Magic Moment:

Daily
Plan

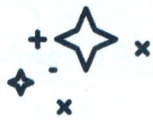

Day at a glance

Remember This!

6 am	
7 am	
8 am	
9 am	
10 am	
11 am	
12 pm	
1 pm	
2 pm	
3 pm	
4 pm	
5 pm	
6 pm	
7 pm	

Top Priorities!

Glass of Water Score

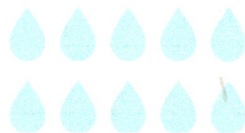

Biggest Learning:

Today's Magic Moment:

Daily
Plan

Remember This!

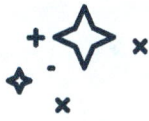

Day at a glance

6 am	
7 am	
8 am	
9 am	
10 am	
11 am	
12 pm	
1 pm	
2 pm	
3 pm	
4 pm	
5 pm	
6 pm	
7 pm	

Top Priorities!

Glass of Water Score

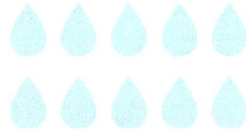

Biggest Learning:

Today's Magic Moment:

Daily

Plan

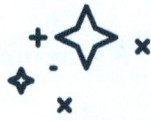

Day at a glance

Time	
6 am	
7 am	
8 am	
9 am	
10 am	
11 am	
12 pm	
1 pm	
2 pm	
3 pm	
4 pm	
5 pm	
6 pm	
7 pm	

Remember This!

Top Priorities!

Glass of Water Score

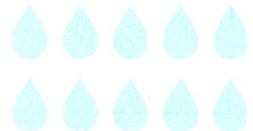

Biggest Learning:

Today's Magic Moment:

Daily Plan

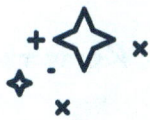

Day at a glance

6 am	
7 am	
8 am	
9 am	
10 am	
11 am	
12 pm	
1 pm	
2 pm	
3 pm	
4 pm	
5 pm	
6 pm	
7 pm	

Top Priorities!

Glass of Water Score

Biggest Learning:

Today's Magic Moment:

Daily
Plan

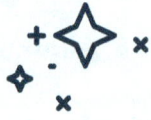

Day at a glance

6 am	
7 am	
8 am	
9 am	
10 am	
11 am	
12 pm	
1 pm	
2 pm	
3 pm	
4 pm	
5 pm	
6 pm	
7 pm	

Top Priorities!

Glass of Water Score

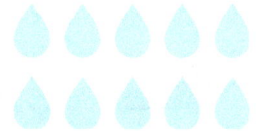

💧💧💧💧💧
💧💧💧💧💧

Biggest Learning:

Today's Magic Moment:

Daily
Plan

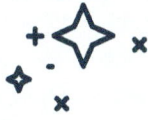

Day at a glance

6 am	
7 am	
8 am	
9 am	
10 am	
11 am	
12 pm	
1 pm	
2 pm	
3 pm	
4 pm	
5 pm	
6 pm	
7 pm	

Remember This!

Top Priorities!

Glass of Water Score

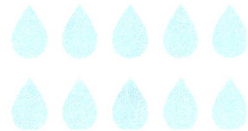

Biggest Learning:

Today's Magic Moment:

Weekly Snapshot

Week Commencing:

New Habit

Name It.

Must Do This Week!

Track It.

- ☐ Mon
- ☐ Tues
- ☐ Wed
- ☐ Thurs
- ☐ Fri
- ☐ Sat
- ☐ Sun

Quote For The Week:

Review It.
How did it go?
What worked?
What didn't?

Daily
Plan

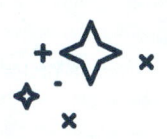

Day at a glance

Remember This!

6 am	
7 am	
8 am	
9 am	
10 am	
11 am	
12 pm	
1 pm	
2 pm	
3 pm	
4 pm	
5 pm	
6 pm	
7 pm	

Top Priorities!

Glass of Water Score

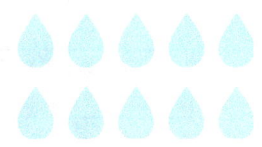

Biggest Learning:

Today's Magic Moment:

Daily Plan

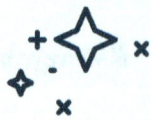

Day at a glance

6 am	
7 am	
8 am	
9 am	
10 am	
11 am	
12 pm	
1 pm	
2 pm	
3 pm	
4 pm	
5 pm	
6 pm	
7 pm	

Remember This!

Top Priorities!

Glass of Water Score

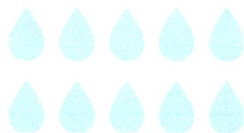

Biggest Learning:

Today's Magic Moment:

Daily

Plan

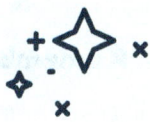

Day at a glance

6 am	
7 am	
8 am	
9 am	
10 am	
11 am	
12 pm	
1 pm	
2 pm	
3 pm	
4 pm	
5 pm	
6 pm	
7 pm	

Remember This!

Top Priorities!

Glass of Water Score

Biggest Learning:

Today's Magic Moment:

Daily Plan

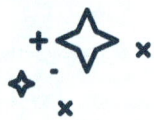

Day at a glance

6 am	
7 am	
8 am	
9 am	
10 am	
11 am	
12 pm	
1 pm	
2 pm	
3 pm	
4 pm	
5 pm	
6 pm	
7 pm	

Top Priorities!

Glass of Water Score

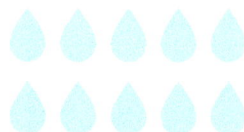

Biggest Learning:

Today's Magic Moment:

Daily Plan

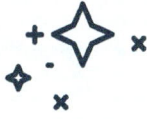

Day at a glance

6 am	
7 am	
8 am	
9 am	
10 am	
11 am	
12 pm	
1 pm	
2 pm	
3 pm	
4 pm	
5 pm	
6 pm	
7 pm	

Remember This!

Top Priorities!

Glass of Water Score

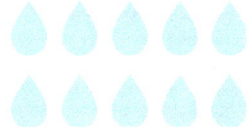

💧💧💧💧💧
💧💧💧💧💧

Biggest Learning:

Today's Magic Moment:

Daily

Plan

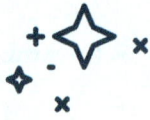

Day at a glance

6 am	
7 am	
8 am	
9 am	
10 am	
11 am	
12 pm	
1 pm	
2 pm	
3 pm	
4 pm	
5 pm	
6 pm	
7 pm	

Remember This!

Top Priorities!

Glass of Water Score

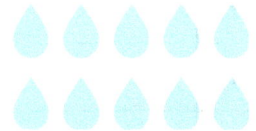

Biggest Learning:

Today's Magic Moment:

Daily Plan

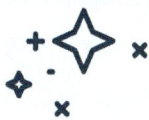

Day at a glance

6 am	
7 am	
8 am	
9 am	
10 am	
11 am	
12 pm	
1 pm	
2 pm	
3 pm	
4 pm	
5 pm	
6 pm	
7 pm	

Remember This!

Top Priorities!

Glass of Water Score

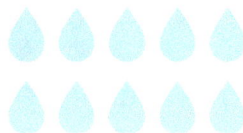

Biggest Learning:

Today's Magic Moment:

Weekly Snapshot

Week Commencing:

Must Do This Week!

New Habit

Name It.

Track It.

- ☐ Mon
- ☐ Tues
- ☐ Wed
- ☐ Thurs
- ☐ Fri
- ☐ Sat
- ☐ Sun

Quote For The Week:

Discipline is the bridge between

goals and accomplishment.

JIM ROHN

Review It.
How did it go?
What worked?
What didn't?

Daily Plan

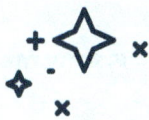

Day at a glance

6 am	
7 am	
8 am	
9 am	
10 am	
11 am	
12 pm	
1 pm	
2 pm	
3 pm	
4 pm	
5 pm	
6 pm	
7 pm	

Remember This!

Top Priorities!

Glass of Water Score

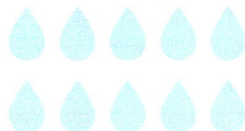

Biggest Learning:

Today's Magic Moment:

Daily

Plan

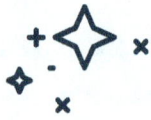

Day at a glance

6 am	
7 am	
8 am	
9 am	
10 am	
11 am	
12 pm	
1 pm	
2 pm	
3 pm	
4 pm	
5 pm	
6 pm	
7 pm	

Top Priorities!

Glass of Water Score

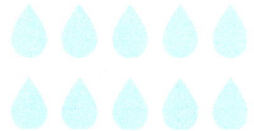

Biggest Learning:

Today's Magic Moment:

Daily Plan

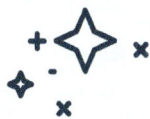

Day at a glance

6 am	
7 am	
8 am	
9 am	
10 am	
11 am	
12 pm	
1 pm	
2 pm	
3 pm	
4 pm	
5 pm	
6 pm	
7 pm	

Remember This!

Top Priorities!

Glass of Water Score

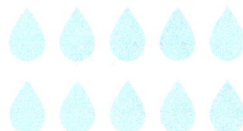

Biggest Learning:

Today's Magic Moment:

Daily Plan

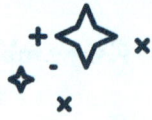

Day at a glance

6 am	
7 am	
8 am	
9 am	
10 am	
11 am	
12 pm	
1 pm	
2 pm	
3 pm	
4 pm	
5 pm	
6 pm	
7 pm	

Remember This!

Top Priorities!

Glass of Water Score

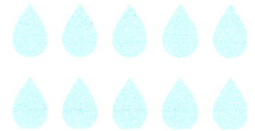

Biggest Learning:

Today's Magic Moment:

Daily Plan

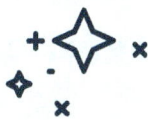

Day at a glance

6 am	
7 am	
8 am	
9 am	
10 am	
11 am	
12 pm	
1 pm	
2 pm	
3 pm	
4 pm	
5 pm	
6 pm	
7 pm	

Remember This!

Top Priorities!

Glass of Water Score

Biggest Learning:

Today's Magic Moment:

Daily Plan

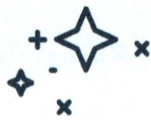

Remember This!

Day at a glance

6 am	
7 am	
8 am	
9 am	
10 am	
11 am	
12 pm	
1 pm	
2 pm	
3 pm	
4 pm	
5 pm	
6 pm	
7 pm	

Top Priorities!

Glass of Water Score

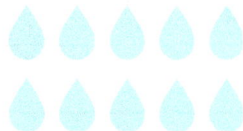

Biggest Learning:

Today's Magic Moment:

Daily
Plan

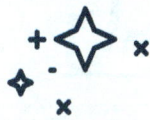

Day at a glance

Remember This!

6 am	
7 am	
8 am	
9 am	
10 am	
11 am	
12 pm	
1 pm	
2 pm	
3 pm	
4 pm	
5 pm	
6 pm	
7 pm	

Top Priorities!

Glass of Water Score

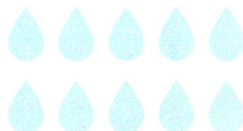

Biggest Learning:

Today's Magic Moment:

Monthly

Focus

Goals	Due By

Tasks

- [ ]
- [ ]
- [ ]
- [ ]
- [ ]
- [ ]

Results

Weekly Snapshot

Week Commencing:

New Habit

Name It.

Must Do This Week!

Track It.

- ☐ Mon
- ☐ Tues
- ☐ Wed
- ☐ Thurs
- ☐ Fri
- ☐ Sat
- ☐ Sun

Quote For The Week:

Rather than mind
the changes of life...
Change your mind
about life.

ISIRA

Review It.
How did it go?
What worked?
What didn't?

Daily
Plan

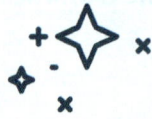

Day at a glance

6 am	
7 am	
8 am	
9 am	
10 am	
11 am	
12 pm	
1 pm	
2 pm	
3 pm	
4 pm	
5 pm	
6 pm	
7 pm	

Remember This!

Top Priorities!

Glass of Water Score

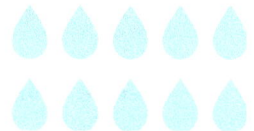

Biggest Learning:

Today's Magic Moment:

Daily Plan

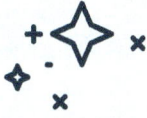

Day at a glance

6 am	
7 am	
8 am	
9 am	
10 am	
11 am	
12 pm	
1 pm	
2 pm	
3 pm	
4 pm	
5 pm	
6 pm	
7 pm	

Remember This!

Top Priorities!

Glass of Water Score

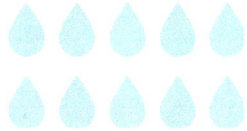

Biggest Learning:

Today's Magic Moment:

Daily Plan

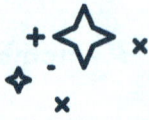

Day at a glance

Remember This!

6 am	
7 am	
8 am	
9 am	
10 am	
11 am	
12 pm	
1 pm	
2 pm	
3 pm	
4 pm	
5 pm	
6 pm	
7 pm	

Top Priorities!

Glass of Water Score

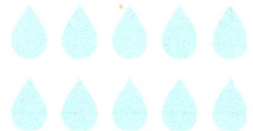

Biggest Learning:

Today's Magic Moment:

Daily Plan

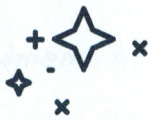

Day at a glance

6 am	
7 am	
8 am	
9 am	
10 am	
11 am	
12 pm	
1 pm	
2 pm	
3 pm	
4 pm	
5 pm	
6 pm	
7 pm	

Remember This!

Top Priorities!

Glass of Water Score

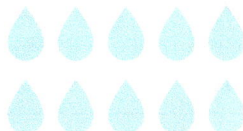

Biggest Learning:

Today's Magic Moment:

Daily Plan

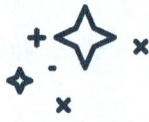

Day at a glance

Time	
6 am	
7 am	
8 am	
9 am	
10 am	
11 am	
12 pm	
1 pm	
2 pm	
3 pm	
4 pm	
5 pm	
6 pm	
7 pm	

Remember This!

Top Priorities!

Glass of Water Score

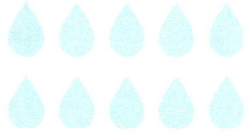

Biggest Learning:

Today's Magic Moment:

Daily Plan

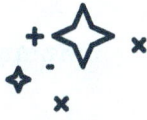

Day at a glance

Time	
6 am	
7 am	
8 am	
9 am	
10 am	
11 am	
12 pm	
1 pm	
2 pm	
3 pm	
4 pm	
5 pm	
6 pm	
7 pm	

Remember This!

Top Priorities!

Glass of Water Score

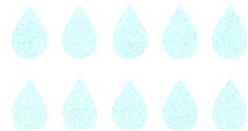

Biggest Learning:

Today's Magic Moment:

Daily Plan

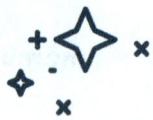

Day at a glance

6 am	
7 am	
8 am	
9 am	
10 am	
11 am	
12 pm	
1 pm	
2 pm	
3 pm	
4 pm	
5 pm	
6 pm	
7 pm	

Remember This!

Top Priorities!

Glass of Water Score

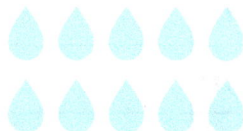

Biggest Learning:

Today's Magic Moment:

Weekly Snapshot

Week Commencing:

New Habit
Name It.

Must Do This Week!

Track It.

- ☐ Mon
- ☐ Tues
- ☐ Wed
- ☐ Thurs
- ☐ Fri
- ☐ Sat
- ☐ Sun

Quote For The Week:

Allow time to daydream, think
and feel what you want.
Wherever the mind has been
the body will follow.

MICHELLE ROBERTSON-JONES

Review It.
How did it go?
What worked?
What didn't?

Daily Plan

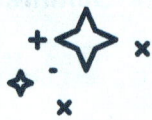

Day at a glance

6 am	
7 am	
8 am	
9 am	
10 am	
11 am	
12 pm	
1 pm	
2 pm	
3 pm	
4 pm	
5 pm	
6 pm	
7 pm	

Remember This!

Top Priorities!

Glass of Water Score

Biggest Learning:

Today's Magic Moment:

Daily Plan

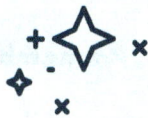

Day at a glance

6 am	
7 am	
8 am	
9 am	
10 am	
11 am	
12 pm	
1 pm	
2 pm	
3 pm	
4 pm	
5 pm	
6 pm	
7 pm	

Remember This!

Top Priorities!

Glass of Water Score

Biggest Learning:

Today's Magic Moment:

Daily Plan

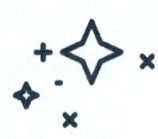

Day at a glance

6 am	
7 am	
8 am	
9 am	
10 am	
11 am	
12 pm	
1 pm	
2 pm	
3 pm	
4 pm	
5 pm	
6 pm	
7 pm	

Remember This!

Top Priorities!

Glass of Water Score

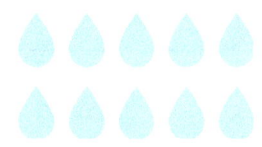

Biggest Learning:

Today's Magic Moment:

Daily Plan

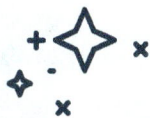

Day at a glance

6 am	
7 am	
8 am	
9 am	
10 am	
11 am	
12 pm	
1 pm	
2 pm	
3 pm	
4 pm	
5 pm	
6 pm	
7 pm	

Remember This!

Top Priorities!

Glass of Water Score

Biggest Learning:

Today's Magic Moment:

Daily Plan

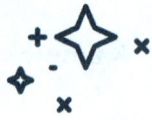

Day at a glance

6 am	
7 am	
8 am	
9 am	
10 am	
11 am	
12 pm	
1 pm	
2 pm	
3 pm	
4 pm	
5 pm	
6 pm	
7 pm	

Remember This!

Top Priorities!

Glass of Water Score

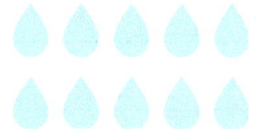

Biggest Learning:

Today's Magic Moment:

Daily Plan

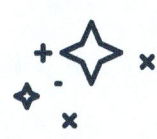

Day at a glance

Time	
6 am	
7 am	
8 am	
9 am	
10 am	
11 am	
12 pm	
1 pm	
2 pm	
3 pm	
4 pm	
5 pm	
6 pm	
7 pm	

Top Priorities!

Glass of Water Score

💧💧💧💧💧
💧💧💧💧💧

Biggest Learning:

Today's Magic Moment:

Daily
Plan

Day at a glance

6 am	
7 am	
8 am	
9 am	
10 am	
11 am	
12 pm	
1 pm	
2 pm	
3 pm	
4 pm	
5 pm	
6 pm	
7 pm	

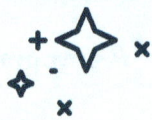

Remember This!

Top Priorities!

Glass of Water Score

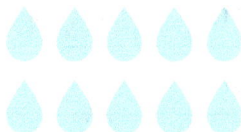

Biggest Learning:

Today's Magic Moment:

Weekly
Snapshot

Week Commencing:

New Habit

Name It.

Must Do This Week!

Track It.

☐ Mon

☐ Tues

☐ Wed

☐ Thurs

☐ Fri

☐ Sat

☐ Sun

Quote For The Week:

Review It.
How did it go?
What worked?
What didn't?

Daily Plan

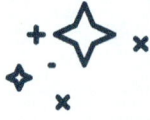

Day at a glance

Time	
6 am	
7 am	
8 am	
9 am	
10 am	
11 am	
12 pm	
1 pm	
2 pm	
3 pm	
4 pm	
5 pm	
6 pm	
7 pm	

Remember This!

Top Priorities!

Glass of Water Score

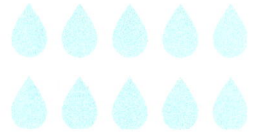

Biggest Learning:

Today's Magic Moment:

Daily Plan

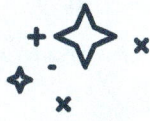

Day at a glance

6 am	
7 am	
8 am	
9 am	
10 am	
11 am	
12 pm	
1 pm	
2 pm	
3 pm	
4 pm	
5 pm	
6 pm	
7 pm	

Remember This!

Top Priorities!

Glass of Water Score

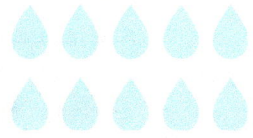

Biggest Learning:

Today's Magic Moment:

Daily Plan

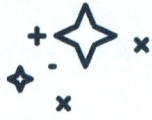

Day at a glance

6 am	
7 am	
8 am	
9 am	
10 am	
11 am	
12 pm	
1 pm	
2 pm	
3 pm	
4 pm	
5 pm	
6 pm	
7 pm	

Remember This!

Top Priorities!

Glass of Water Score

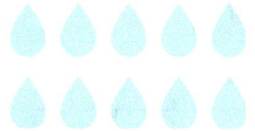

Biggest Learning:

Today's Magic Moment:

Daily Plan

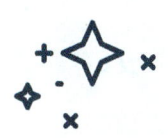

Day at a glance

6 am	
7 am	
8 am	
9 am	
10 am	
11 am	
12 pm	
1 pm	
2 pm	
3 pm	
4 pm	
5 pm	
6 pm	
7 pm	

Remember This!

Top Priorities!

Glass of Water Score

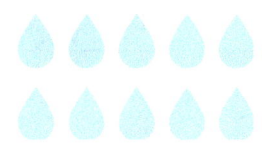

Biggest Learning:

Today's Magic Moment:

Daily
Plan

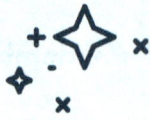

Day at a glance

6 am	
7 am	
8 am	
9 am	
10 am	
11 am	
12 pm	
1 pm	
2 pm	
3 pm	
4 pm	
5 pm	
6 pm	
7 pm	

Top Priorities!

Glass of Water Score

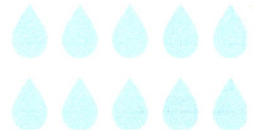

💧💧💧💧💧
💧💧💧💧💧

Biggest Learning:

Today's Magic Moment:

Daily
Plan

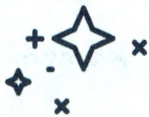

Day at a glance

Remember This!

6 am	
7 am	
8 am	
9 am	
10 am	
11 am	
12 pm	
1 pm	
2 pm	
3 pm	
4 pm	
5 pm	
6 pm	
7 pm	

Top Priorities!

Glass of Water Score

Biggest Learning:

Today's Magic Moment:

Daily
Plan

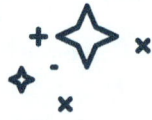

Day at a glance

Remember This!

6 am	
7 am	
8 am	
9 am	
10 am	
11 am	
12 pm	
1 pm	
2 pm	
3 pm	
4 pm	
5 pm	
6 pm	
7 pm	

Top Priorities!

Glass of Water Score

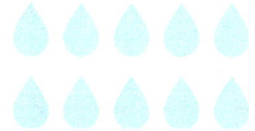

Biggest Learning:

Today's Magic Moment:

Weekly Snapshot

Week Commencing:

New Habit

Name It.

Must Do This Week!

Track It.

☐ Mon

☐ Tues

☐ Wed

☐ Thurs

☐ Fri

☐ Sat

☐ Sun

Quote For The Week:

The best preparation
for tomorrow
is doing your best today.

H. JACKSON BROWN, JR.

Review It.
How did it go?
What worked?
What didn't?

Daily Plan

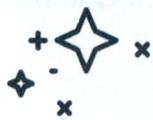

Day at a glance

6 am	
7 am	
8 am	
9 am	
10 am	
11 am	
12 pm	
1 pm	
2 pm	
3 pm	
4 pm	
5 pm	
6 pm	
7 pm	

Remember This!

Top Priorities!

Glass of Water Score

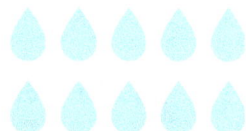

Biggest Learning:

Today's Magic Moment:

Daily Plan

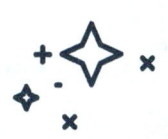

Day at a glance

Time	
6 am	
7 am	
8 am	
9 am	
10 am	
11 am	
12 pm	
1 pm	
2 pm	
3 pm	
4 pm	
5 pm	
6 pm	
7 pm	

Remember This!

Top Priorities!

Glass of Water Score

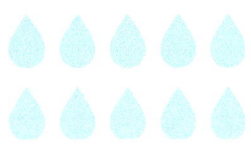

Biggest Learning:

Today's Magic Moment:

Daily Plan

Remember This! ☝️

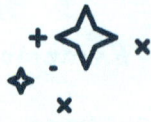

Day at a glance

6 am	
7 am	
8 am	
9 am	
10 am	
11 am	
12 pm	
1 pm	
2 pm	
3 pm	
4 pm	
5 pm	
6 pm	
7 pm	

Top Priorities!

Glass of Water Score

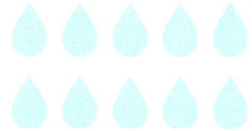

💧💧💧💧💧
💧💧💧💧💧

Biggest Learning:

Today's Magic Moment:

Daily
Plan

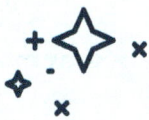

Day at a glance

6 am	
7 am	
8 am	
9 am	
10 am	
11 am	
12 pm	
1 pm	
2 pm	
3 pm	
4 pm	
5 pm	
6 pm	
7 pm	

Remember This!

Top Priorities!

Glass of Water Score

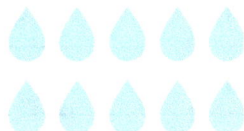

Biggest Learning:

Today's Magic Moment:

Daily
Plan

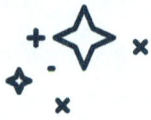

Day at a glance

6 am	
7 am	
8 am	
9 am	
10 am	
11 am	
12 pm	
1 pm	
2 pm	
3 pm	
4 pm	
5 pm	
6 pm	
7 pm	

Top Priorities!

Glass of Water Score

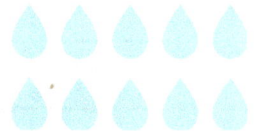

Biggest Learning:

Today's Magic Moment:

Daily Plan

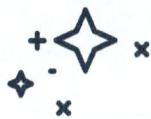

Day at a glance

6 am	
7 am	
8 am	
9 am	
10 am	
11 am	
12 pm	
1 pm	
2 pm	
3 pm	
4 pm	
5 pm	
6 pm	
7 pm	

Remember This!

Top Priorities!

Glass of Water Score

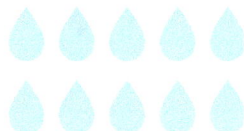

Biggest Learning:

Today's Magic Moment:

Daily Plan

Day at a glance

6 am	
7 am	
8 am	
9 am	
10 am	
11 am	
12 pm	
1 pm	
2 pm	
3 pm	
4 pm	
5 pm	
6 pm	
7 pm	

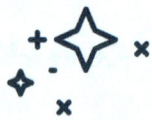

Remember This!

Top Priorities!

Glass of Water Score

Biggest Learning:

Today's Magic Moment:

Weekly Snapshot

Week Commencing:

Must Do This Week!

New Habit

Name It.

Track It.

- ☐ Mon
- ☐ Tues
- ☐ Wed
- ☐ Thurs
- ☐ Fri
- ☐ Sat
- ☐ Sun

Quote For The Week:

Review It.
How did it go?
What worked?
What didn't?

Daily
Plan

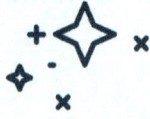

Day at a glance

6 am	
7 am	
8 am	
9 am	
10 am	
11 am	
12 pm	
1 pm	
2 pm	
3 pm	
4 pm	
5 pm	
6 pm	
7 pm	

Top Priorities!

Glass of Water Score

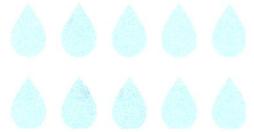

Biggest Learning:

Today's Magic Moment:

Daily Plan

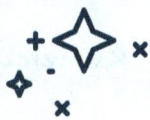

Day at a glance

6 am	
7 am	
8 am	
9 am	
10 am	
11 am	
12 pm	
1 pm	
2 pm	
3 pm	
4 pm	
5 pm	
6 pm	
7 pm	

Remember This!

Top Priorities!

Glass of Water Score

Biggest Learning:

Today's Magic Moment:

Daily Plan

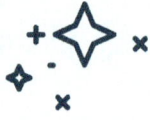

Day at a glance

6 am	
7 am	
8 am	
9 am	
10 am	
11 am	
12 pm	
1 pm	
2 pm	
3 pm	
4 pm	
5 pm	
6 pm	
7 pm	

Top Priorities!

Glass of Water Score

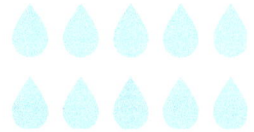

Biggest Learning:

Today's Magic Moment:

Daily Plan

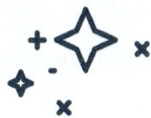

Day at a glance

6 am	
7 am	
8 am	
9 am	
10 am	
11 am	
12 pm	
1 pm	
2 pm	
3 pm	
4 pm	
5 pm	
6 pm	
7 pm	

Remember This!

Top Priorities!

Glass of Water Score

Biggest Learning:

Today's Magic Moment:

Daily
Plan

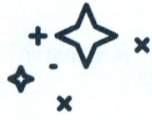

Day at a glance

6 am	
7 am	
8 am	
9 am	
10 am	
11 am	
12 pm	
1 pm	
2 pm	
3 pm	
4 pm	
5 pm	
6 pm	
7 pm	

Remember This!

Top Priorities!

Glass of Water Score

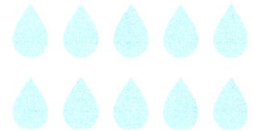

Biggest Learning:

Today's Magic Moment:

Daily
Plan

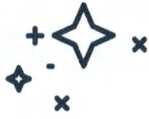

Day at a glance

6 am	
7 am	
8 am	
9 am	
10 am	
11 am	
12 pm	
1 pm	
2 pm	
3 pm	
4 pm	
5 pm	
6 pm	
7 pm	

Remember This!

Top Priorities!

Glass of Water Score

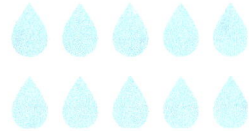

Biggest Learning:

Today's Magic Moment:

Daily Plan

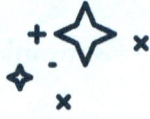

Day at a glance

6 am	
7 am	
8 am	
9 am	
10 am	
11 am	
12 pm	
1 pm	
2 pm	
3 pm	
4 pm	
5 pm	
6 pm	
7 pm	

Top Priorities!

Glass of Water Score

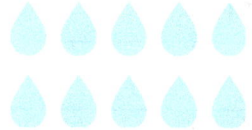

Biggest Learning:

Today's Magic Moment:

Monthly

Focus

Goals	Due By

Tasks

- [ ]
- [ ]
- [ ]
- [ ]
- [ ]
- [ ]

Results

Weekly
Snapshot

New Habit

Name It.

Must Do This Week!

Track It.

- ☐ Mon
- ☐ Tues
- ☐ Wed
- ☐ Thurs
- ☐ Fri
- ☐ Sat
- ☐ Sun

Quote For The Week:

You may have to fight a
battle more than
once to win it.

MARGARET THATCHER

Review It.
How did it go?
What worked?
What didn't?

Daily Plan

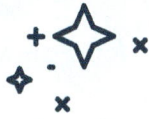

Day at a glance

Time	
6 am	
7 am	
8 am	
9 am	
10 am	
11 am	
12 pm	
1 pm	
2 pm	
3 pm	
4 pm	
5 pm	
6 pm	
7 pm	

Remember This!

Top Priorities!

Glass of Water Score

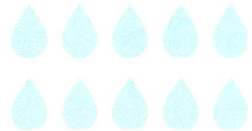

Biggest Learning:

Today's Magic Moment:

Daily Plan

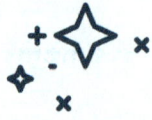

Day at a glance

Time	
6 am	
7 am	
8 am	
9 am	
10 am	
11 am	
12 pm	
1 pm	
2 pm	
3 pm	
4 pm	
5 pm	
6 pm	
7 pm	

Top Priorities!

Glass of Water Score

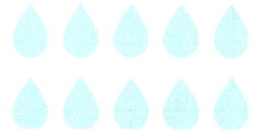

Biggest Learning:

Today's Magic Moment:

Daily Plan

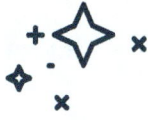

Day at a glance

Remember This!

6 am	
7 am	
8 am	
9 am	
10 am	
11 am	
12 pm	
1 pm	
2 pm	
3 pm	
4 pm	
5 pm	
6 pm	
7 pm	

Top Priorities!

Glass of Water Score

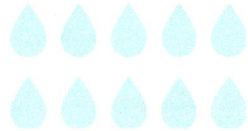

Biggest Learning:

Today's Magic Moment:

Daily Plan

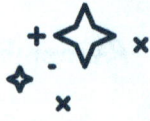

Day at a glance

Remember This!

6 am	
7 am	
8 am	
9 am	
10 am	
11 am	
12 pm	
1 pm	
2 pm	
3 pm	
4 pm	
5 pm	
6 pm	
7 pm	

Top Priorities!

Glass of Water Score

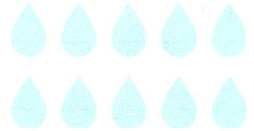

Biggest Learning:

Today's Magic Moment:

Daily Plan

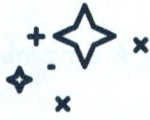

Day at a glance

Time	
6 am	
7 am	
8 am	
9 am	
10 am	
11 am	
12 pm	
1 pm	
2 pm	
3 pm	
4 pm	
5 pm	
6 pm	
7 pm	

Remember This!

Top Priorities!

Glass of Water Score

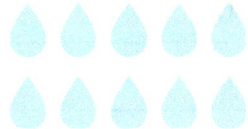

Biggest Learning:

Today's Magic Moment:

Daily

Plan

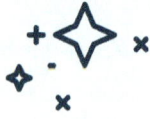

Day at a glance

6 am	
7 am	
8 am	
9 am	
10 am	
11 am	
12 pm	
1 pm	
2 pm	
3 pm	
4 pm	
5 pm	
6 pm	
7 pm	

Remember This!

Top Priorities!

Glass of Water Score

Biggest Learning:

Today's Magic Moment:

Daily Plan

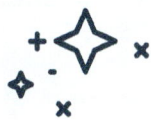

Day at a glance

6 am	
7 am	
8 am	
9 am	
10 am	
11 am	
12 pm	
1 pm	
2 pm	
3 pm	
4 pm	
5 pm	
6 pm	
7 pm	

Remember This!

Top Priorities!

Glass of Water Score

Biggest Learning:

Today's Magic Moment:

Weekly Snapshot

New Habit

Name It.

Must Do This Week!

Track It.

- ☐ Mon
- ☐ Tues
- ☐ Wed
- ☐ Thurs
- ☐ Fri
- ☐ Sat
- ☐ Sun

Quote For The Week:

Every great dream begins

with a dreamer.

Always remember, you have within
you the strength,

the patience, and the passion to

reach for the stars to change

the world.

HARRIET TUBMAN

Review It.

How did it go?
What worked?
What didn't?

Daily
Plan

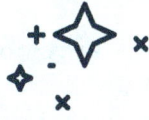

Day at a glance

6 am	
7 am	
8 am	
9 am	
10 am	
11 am	
12 pm	
1 pm	
2 pm	
3 pm	
4 pm	
5 pm	
6 pm	
7 pm	

Remember This!

Top Priorities!

Glass of Water Score

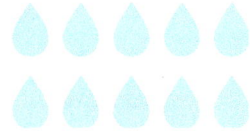

Biggest Learning:

Today's Magic Moment:

Daily Plan

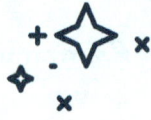

Day at a glance

6 am	
7 am	
8 am	
9 am	
10 am	
11 am	
12 pm	
1 pm	
2 pm	
3 pm	
4 pm	
5 pm	
6 pm	
7 pm	

Remember This!

Top Priorities!

Glass of Water Score

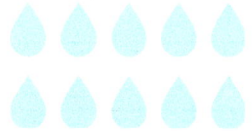

Biggest Learning:

Today's Magic Moment:

Daily Plan

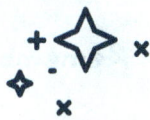

Day at a glance

6 am	
7 am	
8 am	
9 am	
10 am	
11 am	
12 pm	
1 pm	
2 pm	
3 pm	
4 pm	
5 pm	
6 pm	
7 pm	

Remember This!

Top Priorities!

Glass of Water Score

Biggest Learning:

Today's Magic Moment:

Daily
Plan

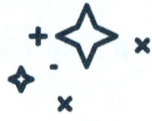

Day at a glance

6 am	
7 am	
8 am	
9 am	
10 am	
11 am	
12 pm	
1 pm	
2 pm	
3 pm	
4 pm	
5 pm	
6 pm	
7 pm	

Top Priorities!

Glass of Water Score

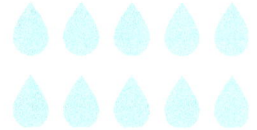

Biggest Learning:

Today's Magic Moment:

Daily Plan

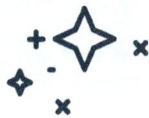

Day at a glance

6 am	
7 am	
8 am	
9 am	
10 am	
11 am	
12 pm	
1 pm	
2 pm	
3 pm	
4 pm	
5 pm	
6 pm	
7 pm	

Remember This!

Top Priorities!

Glass of Water Score

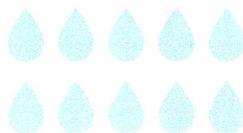

Biggest Learning:

Today's Magic Moment:

Daily Plan

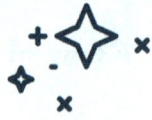

Day at a glance

6 am	
7 am	
8 am	
9 am	
10 am	
11 am	
12 pm	
1 pm	
2 pm	
3 pm	
4 pm	
5 pm	
6 pm	
7 pm	

Remember This!

Top Priorities!

Glass of Water Score

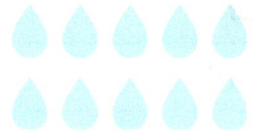

Biggest Learning:

Today's Magic Moment:

Daily Plan

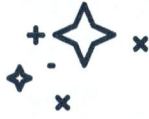

Day at a glance

6 am	
7 am	
8 am	
9 am	
10 am	
11 am	
12 pm	
1 pm	
2 pm	
3 pm	
4 pm	
5 pm	
6 pm	
7 pm	

Remember This!

Top Priorities!

Glass of Water Score

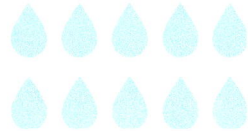

Biggest Learning:

Today's Magic Moment:

Weekly Snapshot

Week Commencing:

Must Do This Week!

_____

_____

_____

_____

_____

_____

Quote For The Week:

New Habit

Name It.

Track It.

- ☐ Mon
- ☐ Tues
- ☐ Wed
- ☐ Thurs
- ☐ Fri
- ☐ Sat
- ☐ Sun

Review It.
How did it go?
What worked?
What didn't?

Daily
Plan

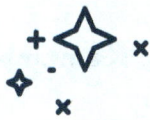

Day at a glance

6 am	
7 am	
8 am	
9 am	
10 am	
11 am	
12 pm	
1 pm	
2 pm	
3 pm	
4 pm	
5 pm	
6 pm	
7 pm	

Top Priorities!

Glass of Water Score

💧💧💧💧💧
💧💧💧💧💧

Biggest Learning:

Today's Magic Moment:

Daily Plan

Day at a glance

6 am	
7 am	
8 am	
9 am	
10 am	
11 am	
12 pm	
1 pm	
2 pm	
3 pm	
4 pm	
5 pm	
6 pm	
7 pm	

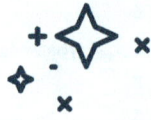

Remember This!

Top Priorities!

Glass of Water Score

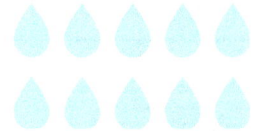

Biggest Learning:

Today's Magic Moment:

Daily
Plan

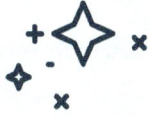

Day at a glance

Time	
6 am	
7 am	
8 am	
9 am	
10 am	
11 am	
12 pm	
1 pm	
2 pm	
3 pm	
4 pm	
5 pm	
6 pm	
7 pm	

Top Priorities!

Glass of Water Score

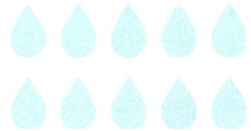

💧💧💧💧💧
💧💧💧💧💧

Biggest Learning:

Today's Magic Moment:

Daily Plan

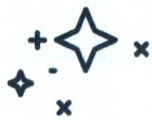

Day at a glance

6 am	
7 am	
8 am	
9 am	
10 am	
11 am	
12 pm	
1 pm	
2 pm	
3 pm	
4 pm	
5 pm	
6 pm	
7 pm	

Remember This!

Top Priorities!

Glass of Water Score

Biggest Learning:

Today's Magic Moment:

Daily
Plan

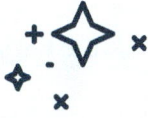

Day at a glance

6 am	
7 am	
8 am	
9 am	
10 am	
11 am	
12 pm	
1 pm	
2 pm	
3 pm	
4 pm	
5 pm	
6 pm	
7 pm	

Remember This!

Top Priorities!

Glass of Water Score

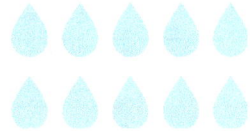

Biggest Learning:

Today's Magic Moment:

Daily Plan

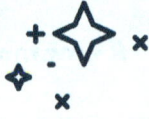

Day at a glance

6 am	
7 am	
8 am	
9 am	
10 am	
11 am	
12 pm	
1 pm	
2 pm	
3 pm	
4 pm	
5 pm	
6 pm	
7 pm	

Remember This!

Top Priorities!

Glass of Water Score

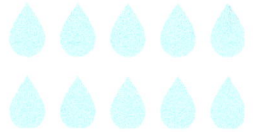

Biggest Learning:

Today's Magic Moment:

Daily Plan

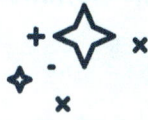

Day at a glance

Time	
6 am	
7 am	
8 am	
9 am	
10 am	
11 am	
12 pm	
1 pm	
2 pm	
3 pm	
4 pm	
5 pm	
6 pm	
7 pm	

Remember This!

Top Priorities!

Glass of Water Score

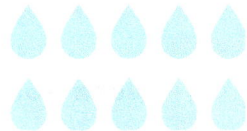

Biggest Learning:

Today's Magic Moment:

Weekly Snapshot

Week Commencing:

Must Do This Week!

New Habit

Name It.

Track It.

- ☐ Mon
- ☐ Tues
- ☐ Wed
- ☐ Thurs
- ☐ Fri
- ☐ Sat
- ☐ Sun

Quote For The Week:

Truth does not become more true by virtue of the fact that the entire world agrees with it, nor less so even if the whole world disagrees with it.

MAIMONIDES

Review It.
How did it go?
What worked?
What didn't?

Daily Plan

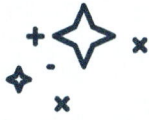

Day at a glance

6 am	
7 am	
8 am	
9 am	
10 am	
11 am	
12 pm	
1 pm	
2 pm	
3 pm	
4 pm	
5 pm	
6 pm	
7 pm	

Remember This!

Top Priorities!

Glass of Water Score

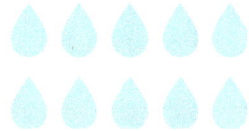

Biggest Learning:

Today's Magic Moment:

Daily Plan

Day at a glance

Time	
6 am	
7 am	
8 am	
9 am	
10 am	
11 am	
12 pm	
1 pm	
2 pm	
3 pm	
4 pm	
5 pm	
6 pm	
7 pm	

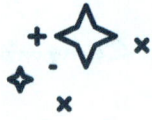

Remember This!

Top Priorities!

Glass of Water Score

Biggest Learning:

Today's Magic Moment:

Daily
Plan

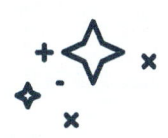

Day at a glance

6 am	
7 am	
8 am	
9 am	
10 am	
11 am	
12 pm	
1 pm	
2 pm	
3 pm	
4 pm	
5 pm	
6 pm	
7 pm	

Remember This!

Top Priorities!

Glass of Water Score

Biggest Learning:

Today's Magic Moment:

Daily Plan

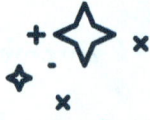

Day at a glance

6 am	
7 am	
8 am	
9 am	
10 am	
11 am	
12 pm	
1 pm	
2 pm	
3 pm	
4 pm	
5 pm	
6 pm	
7 pm	

Top Priorities!

Glass of Water Score

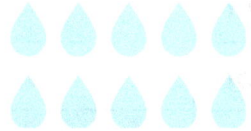

Biggest Learning:

Today's Magic Moment:

Daily Plan

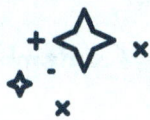

Day at a glance

Time	
6 am	
7 am	
8 am	
9 am	
10 am	
11 am	
12 pm	
1 pm	
2 pm	
3 pm	
4 pm	
5 pm	
6 pm	
7 pm	

Remember This!

Top Priorities!

Glass of Water Score

Biggest Learning:

Today's Magic Moment:

Daily Plan

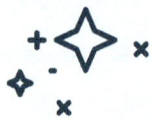

Day at a glance

6 am	
7 am	
8 am	
9 am	
10 am	
11 am	
12 pm	
1 pm	
2 pm	
3 pm	
4 pm	
5 pm	
6 pm	
7 pm	

Remember This!

Top Priorities!

Glass of Water Score

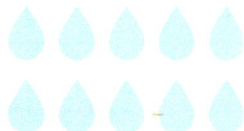

Biggest Learning:

Today's Magic Moment:

Daily Plan

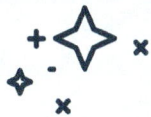

Day at a glance

6 am	
7 am	
8 am	
9 am	
10 am	
11 am	
12 pm	
1 pm	
2 pm	
3 pm	
4 pm	
5 pm	
6 pm	
7 pm	

Remember This!

Top Priorities!

Glass of Water Score

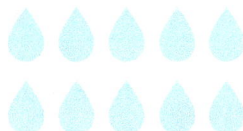

Biggest Learning:

Today's Magic Moment:

Weekly Snapshot

Week Commencing:

New Habit

Name It.

Must Do This Week!

Track It.

- ☐ Mon
- ☐ Tues
- ☐ Wed
- ☐ Thurs
- ☐ Fri
- ☐ Sat
- ☐ Sun

Quote For The Week:

Review It.
How did it go?
What worked?
What didn't?

Daily
Plan

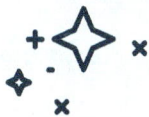

Day at a glance

6 am	
7 am	
8 am	
9 am	
10 am	
11 am	
12 pm	
1 pm	
2 pm	
3 pm	
4 pm	
5 pm	
6 pm	
7 pm	

Top Priorities!

Glass of Water Score

Biggest Learning:

Today's Magic Moment:

Daily Plan

Day at a glance

6 am	
7 am	
8 am	
9 am	
10 am	
11 am	
12 pm	
1 pm	
2 pm	
3 pm	
4 pm	
5 pm	
6 pm	
7 pm	

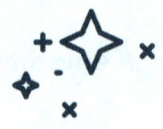

Remember This!

Top Priorities!

Glass of Water Score

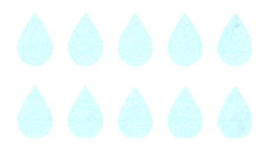

Biggest Learning:

Today's Magic Moment:

Daily
Plan

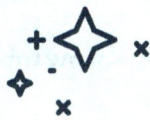

Day at a glance

6 am	
7 am	
8 am	
9 am	
10 am	
11 am	
12 pm	
1 pm	
2 pm	
3 pm	
4 pm	
5 pm	
6 pm	
7 pm	

Remember This!

Top Priorities!

Glass of Water Score

Biggest Learning:

Today's Magic Moment:

Daily
Plan

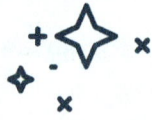

Day at a glance

6 am	
7 am	
8 am	
9 am	
10 am	
11 am	
12 pm	
1 pm	
2 pm	
3 pm	
4 pm	
5 pm	
6 pm	
7 pm	

Top Priorities!

Glass of Water Score

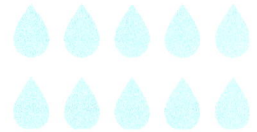

Biggest Learning:

Today's Magic Moment:

Daily Plan

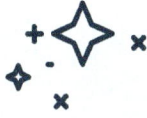

Day at a glance

6 am	
7 am	
8 am	
9 am	
10 am	
11 am	
12 pm	
1 pm	
2 pm	
3 pm	
4 pm	
5 pm	
6 pm	
7 pm	

Remember This!

Top Priorities!

Glass of Water Score

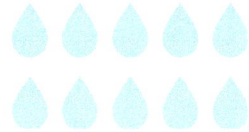

Biggest Learning:

Today's Magic Moment:

Daily Plan

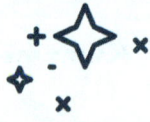

Day at a glance

Time	
6 am	
7 am	
8 am	
9 am	
10 am	
11 am	
12 pm	
1 pm	
2 pm	
3 pm	
4 pm	
5 pm	
6 pm	
7 pm	

Remember This!

Top Priorities!

Glass of Water Score

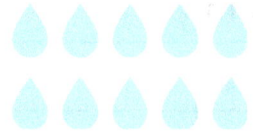

Biggest Learning:

Today's Magic Moment:

Daily Plan

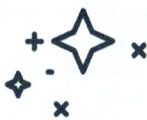

Day at a glance

6 am	
7 am	
8 am	
9 am	
10 am	
11 am	
12 pm	
1 pm	
2 pm	
3 pm	
4 pm	
5 pm	
6 pm	
7 pm	

Remember This!

Top Priorities!

Glass of Water Score

Biggest Learning:

Today's Magic Moment:

Monthly

Focus

Goals	Due By

Results

Tasks

- [ ]
- [ ]
- [ ]
- [ ]
- [ ]
- [ ]

Weekly Snapshot

Week Commencing:

New Habit

Name It.

Must Do This Week!

Track It.

- ☐ Mon
- ☐ Tues
- ☐ Wed
- ☐ Thurs
- ☐ Fri
- ☐ Sat
- ☐ Sun

Quote For The Week:

Review It.
How did it go?
What worked?
What didn't?

Daily
Plan

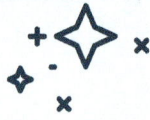

Day at a glance

Remember This!

6 am	
7 am	
8 am	
9 am	
10 am	
11 am	
12 pm	
1 pm	
2 pm	
3 pm	
4 pm	
5 pm	
6 pm	
7 pm	

Top Priorities!

Glass of Water Score

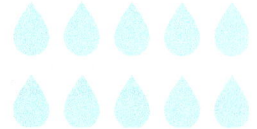

Biggest Learning:

Today's Magic Moment:

Daily Plan

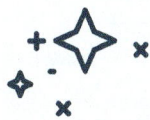

Day at a glance

6 am	
7 am	
8 am	
9 am	
10 am	
11 am	
12 pm	
1 pm	
2 pm	
3 pm	
4 pm	
5 pm	
6 pm	
7 pm	

Remember This!

Top Priorities!

Glass of Water Score

Biggest Learning:

Today's Magic Moment:

Daily
Plan

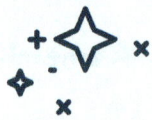

Day at a glance

6 am	
7 am	
8 am	
9 am	
10 am	
11 am	
12 pm	
1 pm	
2 pm	
3 pm	
4 pm	
5 pm	
6 pm	
7 pm	

Top Priorities!

Glass of Water Score

Biggest Learning:

Today's Magic Moment:

Daily Plan

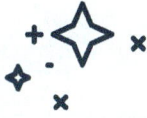

Day at a glance

Remember This!

6 am	
7 am	
8 am	
9 am	
10 am	
11 am	
12 pm	
1 pm	
2 pm	
3 pm	
4 pm	
5 pm	
6 pm	
7 pm	

Top Priorities!

Glass of Water Score

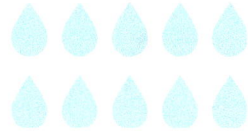

Biggest Learning:

Today's Magic Moment:

Daily Plan

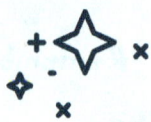

Day at a glance

Time	
6 am	
7 am	
8 am	
9 am	
10 am	
11 am	
12 pm	
1 pm	
2 pm	
3 pm	
4 pm	
5 pm	
6 pm	
7 pm	

Remember This!

Top Priorities!

Glass of Water Score

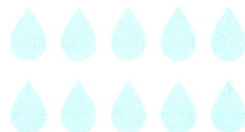

Biggest Learning:

Today's Magic Moment:

Daily Plan

Day at a glance

6 am	
7 am	
8 am	
9 am	
10 am	
11 am	
12 pm	
1 pm	
2 pm	
3 pm	
4 pm	
5 pm	
6 pm	
7 pm	

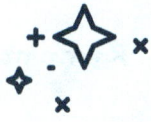

Remember This!

Top Priorities!

Glass of Water Score

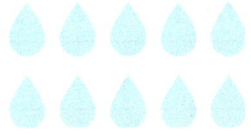

Biggest Learning:

Today's Magic Moment:

Daily
Plan

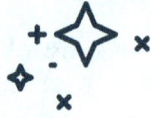

Day at a glance

6 am	
7 am	
8 am	
9 am	
10 am	
11 am	
12 pm	
1 pm	
2 pm	
3 pm	
4 pm	
5 pm	
6 pm	
7 pm	

Top Priorities!

Glass of Water Score

Biggest Learning:

Today's Magic Moment:

Weekly Snapshot

New Habit

Name It.

Must Do This Week!

Track It.

- ☐ Mon
- ☐ Tues
- ☐ Wed
- ☐ Thurs
- ☐ Fri
- ☐ Sat
- ☐ Sun

Quote For The Week:

Things turn out the best
for the people
who make the best out of
the way things turn out
ART LINKLETTER

Review It.
How did it go?
What worked?
What didn't?

Daily Plan

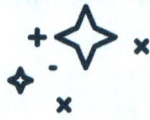

Day at a glance

6 am	
7 am	
8 am	
9 am	
10 am	
11 am	
12 pm	
1 pm	
2 pm	
3 pm	
4 pm	
5 pm	
6 pm	
7 pm	

Remember This!

Top Priorities!

Glass of Water Score

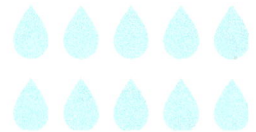

Biggest Learning:

Today's Magic Moment:

Daily Plan

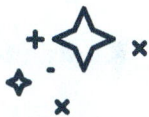

Day at a glance

6 am	
7 am	
8 am	
9 am	
10 am	
11 am	
12 pm	
1 pm	
2 pm	
3 pm	
4 pm	
5 pm	
6 pm	
7 pm	

Remember This!

Top Priorities!

Glass of Water Score

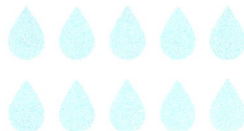

Biggest Learning:

Today's Magic Moment:

Daily Plan

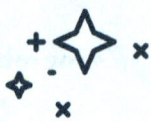

Day at a glance

6 am	
7 am	
8 am	
9 am	
10 am	
11 am	
12 pm	
1 pm	
2 pm	
3 pm	
4 pm	
5 pm	
6 pm	
7 pm	

Remember This!

Top Priorities!

Glass of Water Score

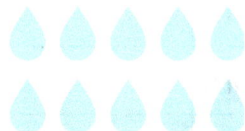

Biggest Learning:

Today's Magic Moment:

Daily Plan

Day at a glance

6 am	
7 am	
8 am	
9 am	
10 am	
11 am	
12 pm	
1 pm	
2 pm	
3 pm	
4 pm	
5 pm	
6 pm	
7 pm	

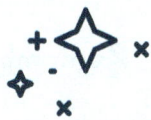

Remember This!

Top Priorities!

Glass of Water Score

Biggest Learning:

Today's Magic Moment:

Daily Plan

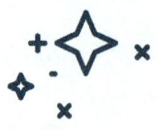

Day at a glance

6 am	
7 am	
8 am	
9 am	
10 am	
11 am	
12 pm	
1 pm	
2 pm	
3 pm	
4 pm	
5 pm	
6 pm	
7 pm	

Remember This!

Top Priorities!

Glass of Water Score

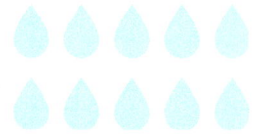

Biggest Learning:

Today's Magic Moment:

Daily
Plan

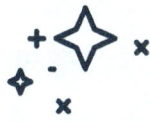

Day at a glance

Remember This!

6 am	
7 am	
8 am	
9 am	
10 am	
11 am	
12 pm	
1 pm	
2 pm	
3 pm	
4 pm	
5 pm	
6 pm	
7 pm	

Top Priorities!

Glass of Water Score

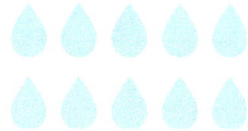

Biggest Learning:

Today's Magic Moment:

Daily Plan

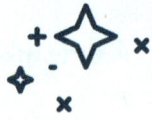

Day at a glance

6 am	
7 am	
8 am	
9 am	
10 am	
11 am	
12 pm	
1 pm	
2 pm	
3 pm	
4 pm	
5 pm	
6 pm	
7 pm	

Remember This!

Top Priorities!

Glass of Water Score

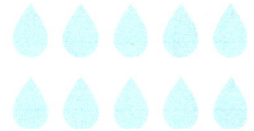

Biggest Learning:

Today's Magic Moment:

Weekly Snapshot

Week Commencing:

New Habit

Name It.

Must Do This Week!

Track It.

- ☐ Mon
- ☐ Tues
- ☐ Wed
- ☐ Thurs
- ☐ Fri
- ☐ Sat
- ☐ Sun

Quote For The Week:

Nothing is difficult
when you break it down
into small pieces.

HENRY FORD

Review It.
How did it go?
What worked?
What didn't?

Daily Plan

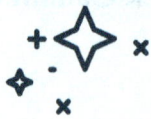

Day at a glance

6 am	
7 am	
8 am	
9 am	
10 am	
11 am	
12 pm	
1 pm	
2 pm	
3 pm	
4 pm	
5 pm	
6 pm	
7 pm	

Remember This!

Top Priorities!

Glass of Water Score

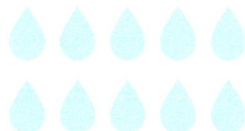

Biggest Learning:

Today's Magic Moment:

Daily Plan

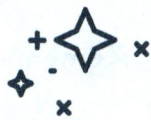

Day at a glance

6 am	
7 am	
8 am	
9 am	
10 am	
11 am	
12 pm	
1 pm	
2 pm	
3 pm	
4 pm	
5 pm	
6 pm	
7 pm	

Remember This!

Top Priorities!

Glass of Water Score

Biggest Learning:

Today's Magic Moment:

Daily
Plan

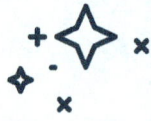

Day at a glance

6 am	
7 am	
8 am	
9 am	
10 am	
11 am	
12 pm	
1 pm	
2 pm	
3 pm	
4 pm	
5 pm	
6 pm	
7 pm	

Remember This!

Top Priorities!

Glass of Water Score

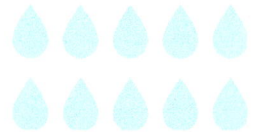

Biggest Learning:

Today's Magic Moment:

Daily Plan

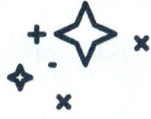

Day at a glance

6 am	
7 am	
8 am	
9 am	
10 am	
11 am	
12 pm	
1 pm	
2 pm	
3 pm	
4 pm	
5 pm	
6 pm	
7 pm	

Top Priorities!

Glass of Water Score

Biggest Learning:

Today's Magic Moment:

Daily Plan

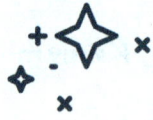

Day at a glance

6 am	
7 am	
8 am	
9 am	
10 am	
11 am	
12 pm	
1 pm	
2 pm	
3 pm	
4 pm	
5 pm	
6 pm	
7 pm	

Remember This!

Top Priorities!

Glass of Water Score

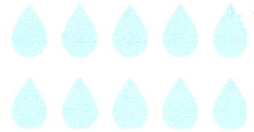

Biggest Learning:

Today's Magic Moment:

Daily
Plan

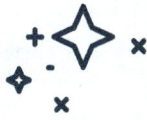

Day at a glance

6 am	
7 am	
8 am	
9 am	
10 am	
11 am	
12 pm	
1 pm	
2 pm	
3 pm	
4 pm	
5 pm	
6 pm	
7 pm	

Top Priorities!

Glass of Water Score

Biggest Learning:

Today's Magic Moment:

Daily Plan

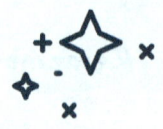

Day at a glance

6 am	
7 am	
8 am	
9 am	
10 am	
11 am	
12 pm	
1 pm	
2 pm	
3 pm	
4 pm	
5 pm	
6 pm	
7 pm	

Remember This!

Top Priorities!

Glass of Water Score

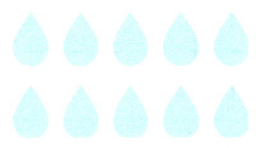

Biggest Learning:

Today's Magic Moment:

Weekly Snapshot

Week Commencing:

New Habit

Name It.

Must Do This Week!

Track It.

- ☐ Mon
- ☐ Tues
- ☐ Wed
- ☐ Thurs
- ☐ Fri
- ☐ Sat
- ☐ Sun

Quote For The Week:

Setting goals is the first step in turning the invisible into the visible!

ANTHONY ROBBINS

Review It.
How did it go?
What worked?
What didn't?

Daily Plan

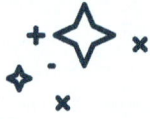

Day at a glance

6 am	
7 am	
8 am	
9 am	
10 am	
11 am	
12 pm	
1 pm	
2 pm	
3 pm	
4 pm	
5 pm	
6 pm	
7 pm	

Remember This!

Top Priorities!

Glass of Water Score

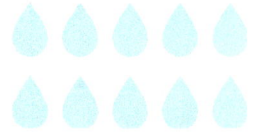

Biggest Learning:

Today's Magic Moment:

Daily Plan

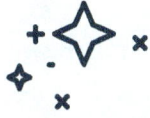

Day at a glance

6 am	
7 am	
8 am	
9 am	
10 am	
11 am	
12 pm	
1 pm	
2 pm	
3 pm	
4 pm	
5 pm	
6 pm	
7 pm	

Top Priorities!

Glass of Water Score

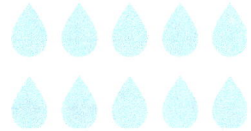

Biggest Learning:

Today's Magic Moment:

Daily Plan

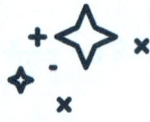

Day at a glance

6 am	
7 am	
8 am	
9 am	
10 am	
11 am	
12 pm	
1 pm	
2 pm	
3 pm	
4 pm	
5 pm	
6 pm	
7 pm	

Remember This!

Top Priorities!

Glass of Water Score

Biggest Learning:

Today's Magic Moment:

Daily Plan

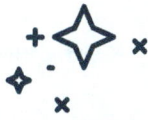

Day at a glance

6 am	
7 am	
8 am	
9 am	
10 am	
11 am	
12 pm	
1 pm	
2 pm	
3 pm	
4 pm	
5 pm	
6 pm	
7 pm	

Top Priorities!

Glass of Water Score

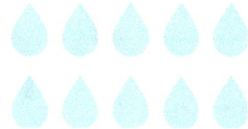

Biggest Learning:

Today's Magic Moment:

Daily Plan

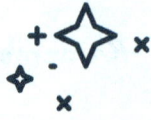

Day at a glance

6 am	
7 am	
8 am	
9 am	
10 am	
11 am	
12 pm	
1 pm	
2 pm	
3 pm	
4 pm	
5 pm	
6 pm	
7 pm	

Remember This!

Top Priorities!

Glass of Water Score

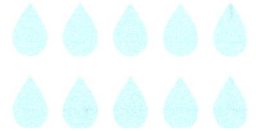

Biggest Learning:

Today's Magic Moment:

Daily Plan

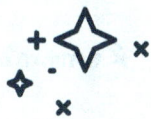

Day at a glance

6 am	
7 am	
8 am	
9 am	
10 am	
11 am	
12 pm	
1 pm	
2 pm	
3 pm	
4 pm	
5 pm	
6 pm	
7 pm	

Remember This!

Top Priorities!

Glass of Water Score

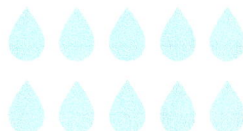

Biggest Learning:

Today's Magic Moment:

Daily Plan

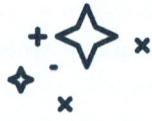

Day at a glance

6 am	
7 am	
8 am	
9 am	
10 am	
11 am	
12 pm	
1 pm	
2 pm	
3 pm	
4 pm	
5 pm	
6 pm	
7 pm	

Remember This!

Top Priorities!

Glass of Water Score

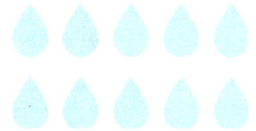

Biggest Learning:

Today's Magic Moment:

Weekly Snapshot

Week Commencing:

New Habit

Name It.

Must Do This Week!

Track It.

- ☐ Mon
- ☐ Tues
- ☐ Wed
- ☐ Thurs
- ☐ Fri
- ☐ Sat
- ☐ Sun

Quote For The Week:

Review It.
How did it go?
What worked?
What didn't?

Daily Plan

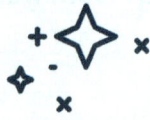

Day at a glance

6 am	
7 am	
8 am	
9 am	
10 am	
11 am	
12 pm	
1 pm	
2 pm	
3 pm	
4 pm	
5 pm	
6 pm	
7 pm	

Remember This!

Top Priorities!

Glass of Water Score

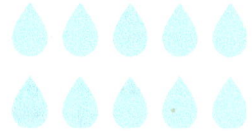

Biggest Learning:

Today's Magic Moment:

Daily Plan

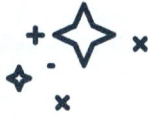

Day at a glance

6 am	
7 am	
8 am	
9 am	
10 am	
11 am	
12 pm	
1 pm	
2 pm	
3 pm	
4 pm	
5 pm	
6 pm	
7 pm	

Top Priorities!

Glass of Water Score

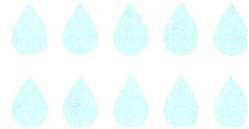

💧💧💧💧💧
💧💧💧💧💧

Biggest Learning:

Today's Magic Moment:

Daily

Plan

Day at a glance

6 am	
7 am	
8 am	
9 am	
10 am	
11 am	
12 pm	
1 pm	
2 pm	
3 pm	
4 pm	
5 pm	
6 pm	
7 pm	

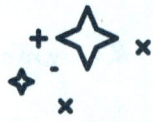

Remember This!

Top Priorities!

Glass of Water Score

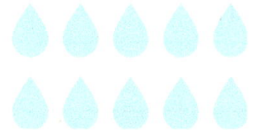

Biggest Learning:

Today's Magic Moment:

Daily
Plan

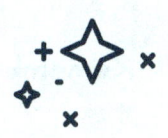

Day at a glance

6 am	
7 am	
8 am	
9 am	
10 am	
11 am	
12 pm	
1 pm	
2 pm	
3 pm	
4 pm	
5 pm	
6 pm	
7 pm	

Top Priorities!

Glass of Water Score

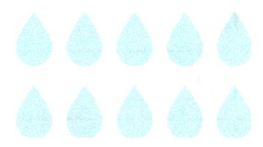

Biggest Learning:

Today's Magic Moment:

Daily
Plan

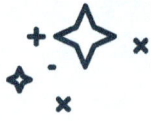

Day at a glance

6 am	
7 am	
8 am	
9 am	
10 am	
11 am	
12 pm	
1 pm	
2 pm	
3 pm	
4 pm	
5 pm	
6 pm	
7 pm	

Remember This!

Top Priorities!

Glass of Water Score

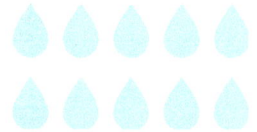

Biggest Learning:

Today's Magic Moment:

Daily Plan

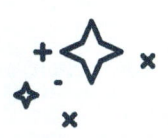

Day at a glance

6 am	
7 am	
8 am	
9 am	
10 am	
11 am	
12 pm	
1 pm	
2 pm	
3 pm	
4 pm	
5 pm	
6 pm	
7 pm	

Remember This!

Top Priorities!

Glass of Water Score

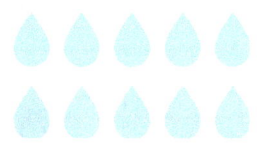

Biggest Learning:

Today's Magic Moment:

Daily Plan

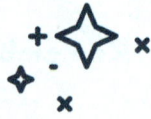

Day at a glance

6 am	
7 am	
8 am	
9 am	
10 am	
11 am	
12 pm	
1 pm	
2 pm	
3 pm	
4 pm	
5 pm	
6 pm	
7 pm	

Remember This!

Top Priorities!

Glass of Water Score

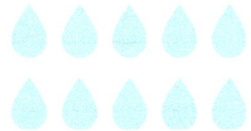

Biggest Learning:

Today's Magic Moment:

Congratulations!

You have made a whole year of progress!

Remember to reward your new self in some way that reflects everything you have achieved throughout the year.

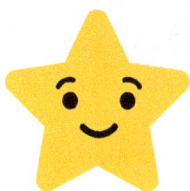

The Big Picture

Now, start on your next goal!

12 Month Planner

January

February

March

April

May

June

July

August

September

October

November

December

Look for our other titles:

Training Tracker

Healthy Habits

Progressive Practice

Happiness Helper

www.ingramcontent.com/pod-product-compliance
Lightning Source LLC
Chambersburg PA
CBHW060018030426
42334CB00019B/2083